Praise for
ShapeWalking

ShapeWalking combines an efficient but simple strength training program with instructions on how to improve your walking style. Improvement of your walking style is a very effective way to keep fit. *ShapeWalking* is not only a useful, but also a pleasant guide for everyone who wants to walk through life healthy! It is top preventive medicine!

— Alex Vaassen, M.D.
Senior Staff Member, Dept. of PhysioTherapie Leiden Medical Center
Leiden, Netherlands

ShapeWalking is a well-thought-out, scientifically based, safe exercise program of moderate intensity. It meets the recommendations of the 1996 *Surgeon General's Report on Physical Activity and Health* for type and quantity of activity per week to promote health.

— Arthur S. Leon, M.D., M.S.
Taylor Professor and director of the Laboratory of Physiological Hygiene
and Exercise Science Division of Kinesiology, University of Minnesota

Bach worked with physical therapist and co-author... Schleck on a program that takes simple walking to new heights of health.

— Audrey DeLaMarte
Steps for Recovery "Book and CD Reviews"
Sherman Oaks, California, February 1999

Exercise is an essential component of an effective psychiatric regimen. I highly recommend *ShapeWalking* to private patients and busy corporate clients. It provides a thorough and effective approach to whole-body health.

— Alfred Messore, M.D.
Washington, DC

ShapeWalking fits into my busy personal and professional schedules. It works for me!

— *Janett Trubatch, Ph.D.*
vice provost for Graduate Studies, Research and Outreach
University of Rhode Island

As a professional businesswoman for an international corporation I am hard-pressed to consistently take exercise classes or join an expensive health club. *ShapeWalking* provides a well-rounded, easy fitness program that I can do at home or when I travel. It's not only fun, it's effective too! It has made a real difference in shaping my thighs especially!

— *Barbara Laska*
Senior Contract Administrator, Ecolab, Inc., St. Paul, MN

Using the techniques and philosophy of *ShapeWalking* I have changed my self-image! By using specific movements described in *ShapeWalking*, my walking routine is now a focused and efficient workout. *ShapeWalking* is ideally suited to my personal-coaching clients who want to add zest to their own exercise routines.

— *Karen J. Carr*
Personal Life Coach carreyes@qwest.net, Vadnais Heights, Minnesota

Since the band [equipment] fits perfectly into my flight bag, I can maintain my exercise schedule during hectic business trips.

— *Joyce Schmidt*
president and CEO of Creative Connections, New London, Connecticut

Today everyone understands the importance of fitness. As a health education consultant, I find *ShapeWalking* a useful tool for helping people enjoy doing what they know is good for them. The sound and easy-to-follow exercises give a balanced focus on both strength and aerobics while allowing the client to concentrate on trouble spots.

— *Janice S. Novak, M.S.*
Health Educator and author of Posture: Get It Straight
www.ImproveYourPosture.com, Eden Prairie, Minnesota

Shape Walking

six easy steps to your best body

Marilyn L. Bach, Ph.D. & Lorie Schleck, M.A., P.T.

BARNES & NOBLE BOOKS

NEW YORK

Fine Communications
322 Eighth Avenue
New York, NY 10001

Shapewalking
LC Control Number 2003115183
ISBN 1-56731-647-6

This special edition published by MJF Books in arrangement with Hunter
House, Inc.

Manufactured in the United States of America on acid-free paper ∞

MJF Books is a trademark of Fine Creative Media, Inc.

QM   10 9 8 7 6 5 4 3

Dedication

This book is dedicated to the women of my family:

To the memory of my mother, Ida, whose regimen of daily walks inspired its writing;

To my sister, Elaine, whose dedication to treadmill walking inspires us all;

To my daughter, Wendy, whose love of dance and Pilates keeps her fit and buff;

To my granddaughter, Maya, who with her joy in gymnastics and ballet will carry forward the family legacy of athleticism.

About the Authors

Marilyn L. Bach, Ph.D.

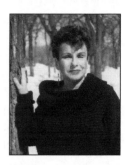

Marilyn L. Bach, Ph.D., is the founder and owner of *Heel to Toe Fitness Walking*, St. Paul, Minnesota, and designer of the *ShapeWalking* program. Dr. Bach, a fitness consultant, is a personal trainer certified by the American Council on Exercise and a member of the American College of Sports Medicine. She has extensive experience as a research scientist/faculty member at several graduate and medical schools, including the Massachusetts Institute of Technology, the University of Wisconsin School of Medicine, and the University of Minnesota Medical School.

Lorie Schleck, M.A., P.T.

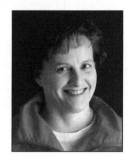

Lorie Schleck, M.A., P.T., physical therapist and fitness consultant, is Director of Physical and Occupational Therapy Continuing Education Home Study Programs for Dogwood Institute, Atlanta, Georgia. She is the author of many health and fitness articles and the book *Staying Strong: A Senior's Guide to a More Independent and Active Life*.

Important Note

The material in this book is intended to provide a safe, effective exercise program. Every effort has been made to provide accurate and dependable information. However, the reader is advised to consult a physician before beginning any exercise program, especially any reader with preexisting medical problems. As health-care professionals have differing opinions and advances in medical and scientific research are made very quickly, the publisher, authors, editors, and professionals quoted in the book cannot be held responsible for any error, omission, dated material, or adverse outcomes that may result from using the information and exercises in this book in a program of self-care or under the care of a licensed practitioner.

If you have questions concerning your exercise program or about the application of the information described in this book, consult a qualified health-care professional.

Contents

Contents

Contents

Acknowledgments

The authors wish to thank the following individuals for technical advice: Arthur Leon, M.D., University of Minnesota; Sandra Swami, R.D., Peggy Struble and Gayle Winegar, The SweatShop, St. Paul, Minnesota; Kate Larson, Winning Lifestyles, Inc., Minneapolis, Minnesota; Terry Wilcox, Resultants for Business, Inc., Hudson, Wisconsin; Glen Carrigan, Progressive Education, Bluffton, South Carolina; and Gwen Hyatt, Desert Southwest Fitness, Inc., Tucson, Arizona.

Special acknowledgments to Mary Beth O'Halloran and Jean Byrne for editing.

Illustrations by Peter Lane, St. Paul, Minnesota. Photography by John Lehn; modeling by Kristin Smith, KAS Fitness Training; graphics by Karla Caspari, Caspari Design Group, all of Minneapolis, Minnesota.

Fitness wardrobe courtesy of Run N Fun, St. Paul, Minnesota.

Foreword

Most of us know that the road to a healthier lifestyle, a smaller waistline, and a firmer body is a one-way street that partners a sound nutritional program with exercise. The medical evidence supporting the benefits of exercise is indisputable. Study after study shows that heart disease, colon cancer, diabetes, osteoporosis, depression, anxiety, and obesity are all significantly less common among those who exercise regularly.

Furthermore, fit people have extra energy and more enthusiasm. They see their lives and futures as positive and hopeful. In fact, if a pill could deliver all the physical and emotional benefits of regular exercise, we would call it a miracle drug.

But beginning and sticking with exercise is much harder than swallowing a pill. As president and owner of Nutritional Weight and Wellness, a center for health-ful nutrition to maximize your health and well-being, I meet clients who have the best intentions, but who often let exercise slack when pressed by the busyness of their schedules. Others work out regularly but then have trouble getting back into their fitness regimen after missing a few weeks while traveling for work or vacation or when pressed for time by busy schedules.

The first edition of *ShapeWalking: Six Easy Steps to a Healthier Life* gave beginners an easy-to-follow, balanced, and well-thought-out program of moderate-intensity exercise. The program begins with walking, a form of exercise that people stick to more than they do any other.

This second edition has all the merits of the earlier version and provides additional guidance for those wishing to shape particular areas of their physique. The program is user-friendly, low-cost, portable, and compliant with the best advice about health benefits.

ShapeWalking is also in compliance with the recommendations of both The American College of Sports Medicine and the 1996 Surgeon General's Report on Physical Activity and Health, so you know you are following a program good for your fitness and for your health.

Exercise truly is the miracle drug. For your best wellness, combine a sound nutritional approach with the superb program of this second edition of *ShapeWalking: Six Easy Steps to Your Best Body*.

— Darlene Kvist, M.S., CNS, L.N.
President and Owner, Nutritional Weight and Wellness
St. Paul, Minnesota

Preface

When meeting fans of the first edition of *ShapeWalking*, I am often asked two questions.

First, "Why have you prepared a second edition of *ShapeWalking*?" Second, "Why do you now give special attention to shaping "trouble spots" such as the abdomen (abs), butt, thighs, and arms?

To answer the first question, we wrote this new edition in response to multiple requests for an updated version of *ShapeWalking*. What could be a better reason to make sure the program stays readily available to the growing number of people who recognize that regular exercise is necessary for health and well-being? In both editions, *ShapeWalking* presents an easy, low-cost, total fitness program based on aerobic walking to burn fat and calories; strengthening exercises to build and tone muscles; and stretching exercises to keep your whole body working smoothly.

The first publication was met with great interest by the general public, the medical profession, and the media, particularly book clubs. *ShapeWalking* was the sole fitness title featured in Health Books Special Edition (Associated Press, 1999). It was three times main selection/editor's choice for Prevention Book Club (Rodale), and it was an alternate selection of the Nurse's Book Society (BookSpan, formerly Doubleday Select). As a result of this high visibility, we received multiple requests for an update. My answer to popular and professional demand: "Here it is!"

In response to the second question—why give special attention to shaping trouble spots such as the abdomen (abs), butt, thighs, and arms—I again defer to public and professional interest. In classes and seminars where I present the *ShapeWalking* program, participants express appreciation for *ShapeWalking's* no-nonsense, no-expensive-equipment portability and ease. But some participants want to go beyond the basic program and attack their individual trouble spots.

This edition answers their request. We have combined Fitness Walking, for an easily accessible aerobic component, with simple Strength Training and stretching exercises (all springing from the first edition), to provide an overall toning program. This edition presents two new sections to help shape your trouble spots. First, Fitness Walking Plus consists of regular Fitness Walking plus shaping components that are performed during your walk to tone your abs, butt, arms, and thighs. Next, Target Toning improves the looks and function of those specially troublesome areas. Those happily using the first edition will surely enjoy the added benefits of this second edition of *ShapeWalking*.

So if you're lumpy and bumpy where you want to be smooth and sleek, or flabby and floppy where you'd rather be tight and toned, welcome to *ShapeWalking*! Just turn the page and get ready to start on your new path to your best body.

— Marilyn L. Bach, Ph.D.
St. Paul, Minnesota

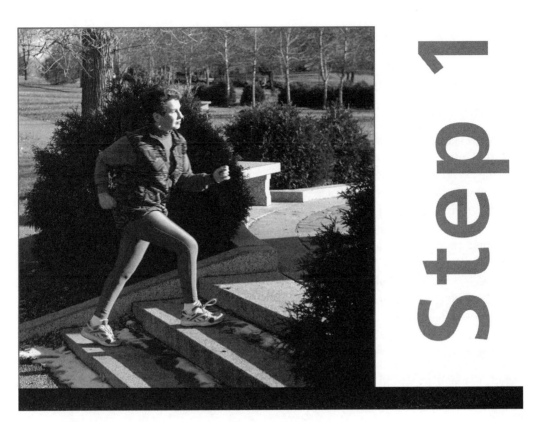

Making the Decision—
Are You Ready to Shape Up
with *ShapeWalking?*

If you're lumpy and bumpy where you want to be smooth and sleek, or flabby and floppy where you'd rather be tight and toned, welcome to *ShapeWalking!*

Step 1: Making the Decision

Why Is *ShapeWalking* Right for Shaping Your Body?

This easy, low-cost program has been designed as a total body-shaping and fitness package. With aerobic exercise to burn fat and calories, strengthening exercises to strengthen and tone your muscles, target toning to attack your trouble spots, and stretching exercises to keep it all working smoothly, *ShapeWalking* has everything you need to get in shape—and improve your shape at the same time.

ShapeWalking is a four-part total fitness program designed to help you achieve your best body:

Fitness Walking: A variation of everyday walking that provides essential aerobic activity.

Fitness Walking Plus: Regular fitness walking plus shaping components that are performed during your walk to tone your abdomen (abs), butt, arms, and thighs.

Strength Training: An overall strength-training program that tones your body's major muscles.

Target Toning (Target muscle/ muscle-group toning): Special bonus toning exercises to turn your trouble spots into a toned abdomen, shapely butt, sleek and more firm "solid" thighs, and firm upper arms.

ShapeWalking starts with Fitness Walking, a variation of ordinary walking, and then adds simple techniques to improve muscle strength and flexibility. The only equipment you will need is a well-designed pair of walking shoes, an exercise band, and some free weights. There are no heavy weights to lift or trendy health clubs to join or new-fangled exercise gadgets to buy. Every component and activity is designed with better body shaping in mind.

ShapeWalking is an extremely versatile program that can be done by anyone, anywhere, any time. It is based on two simple principles: maximum effectiveness and easy accessibility. Based on the newest research and sound scientific principles in the fields of medicine, fitness, and physical therapy, ShapeWalking is done in six steps:

STEP 1: Making the Decision—Are You Ready to Shape Up with *ShapeWalking*

STEP 2: Getting Started with Fitness Walking

STEP 3: Fitness Walking Plus

STEP 4: Strength Training

STEP 5: Target Toning

STEP 6: A Week in the Life of a *ShapeWalker*

These steps will make the most of the time and effort you put into creating a better body shape.

ShapeWalking

A four-part total fitness program designed to help you achieve your best body

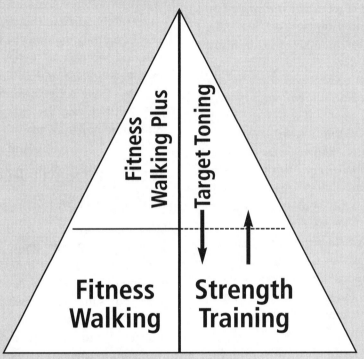

FITNESS WALKING: A variation of everyday walking that provides essential aerobic activity.

FITNESS WALKING PLUS: Regular fitness walking plus shaping components that are performed during your walk to tone your abdomen (abs), butt, arms, and thighs.

STRENGTH TRAINING: An overall strength-training program that tones your body's major muscles.

TARGET TONING: Special bonus toning exercises to shape your trouble spots into a toned abdomen, shapely butt, sleek and solid thighs, and firm upper arms.

What Does a Better Body Shape Mean to You?

As fitness professionals, we are bombarded with specific body-shaping questions. How do I get flat abs? How do I get a shapelier butt? How do I get rid of these saddlebags on my thighs? Our answer: Start *ShapeWalking*!

Deb has a small waist but big hips. Jim is developing a tire around his waist. Sharon has small hips and a flat butt. Marty wants to tone his arms. Amy wants thinner thighs. If there is an ideal body shape out there, very few of us have it. When it comes to the shape of our bodies, we all have strong points and what feel like are glaring weak points. So what can *ShapeWalking* do to improve your shape?

Each of us has a general body shape that is determined by our frame or skeletal system—you may have heard the phrases "big-boned" or "small-framed"—and when you lose weight, you lose fat all over. *ShapeWalking* cannot change your basic body structure or reduce fat in any specific area. No fitness program can.

But *ShapeWalking* can help you lose weight and lower your percentage of body fat. It can tone your muscles so they are firm and strong. And it can help firm-up and thereby improve the shape of trouble areas through target-toning exercises designed to address one specific area.

For example, Christina started the *ShapeWalking* program after her third child. She was interested in getting in shape, but especially concerned with shaping up her flabby stomach. She Fitness Walked, Strength Trained, and Target Toned her abdominal muscles. After three months on the program, she felt better all over and was especially pleased with her improved stomach muscle tone.

What's the secret behind *ShapeWalking*? You. You add the energy and commitment to make it work.

Walking Is Easily Accessible and Low Risk

Most of us learned to walk when we were about a year old. We know how to do it well; in fact, it is second nature to us. So walking is an easy choice for a fitness program that is high on accessibility.

Walking requires only two things: properly fitting shoes and a place to walk —a scenic path, an indoor mall, or a treadmill in bad weather. And Fitness Walking is extremely low risk. The impact on your lower limbs of jogging or running is equivalent to about three times your body weight. (This is partly why running-related injuries are so common.) But the impact of Fitness Walking is only a little over your normal body weight. It's easy to see why fitness experts applaud walking and its low injury risk.

Fitness Walking Is Different from Everyday Walking

Fitness Walking is a special kind of walking. It lends itself to moving faster, working harder, and burning more calories.

Fitness Walking is easy to learn. Almost anyone can do it with a little direction and a bit of practice.

Fitness Walking...

- has a clear form. It emphasizes proper posture, good alignment, and a simple technique.

- sets a faster pace than everyday walking, at 13 to 18 minutes per mile.

- keeps your heart rate in the target zone. The target zone presents the appropriate range (zone) for exercise intensity (how hard you are working). You want to be working hard enough to challenge your body for an effective workout (the lower end of the zone) but not so hard that you overtax your body (the upper end of the zone).

Every time you slip into high gear by changing from ordinary walking to Fitness Walking, you burn more calories and work important muscles harder. In other words, you are shaping up!

Fitness Walking and Weight Loss

For many people, changing body shape is about losing weight and keeping it off.

The only shape they are interested in is a smaller one!

For these people, *ShapeWalking* works great. Fitness Walking burns calories while you walk and increases your metabolism for several hours after your workout. This burns even more calories.

Because Fitness Walking is easy to master, many think it is not real exercise. Don't be fooled. Fitness Walking works major muscle groups. It gets your heart pumping and gets you moving. It does all the things you need to do to lose weight and get in shape. Plus, many studies have found that walking is the one exercise that people tend to stick with the most. Long after the runners have stopped running and the exercise equipment is gathering dust in the basement, walkers are still going strong. And sticking with a program is what helps people not only lose weight, but keep it off.

ShapeWalking adds Strength Training to Fitness Walking for an even more potent weight-loss formula. The stronger and more toned a muscle is, the more calories it burns, even when you are resting. And of course, toned muscles look more sleek and shapely.

Fitness Walking Plus

Once you have Fitness Walking down, we will introduce you to Fitness Walking Plus—fitness walking *plus* a shaping component. You will learn how to walk in a manner that emphasizes use of the abdominal muscles, toning them as you go. You will learn how to add a little buttocks exercise to each step, how to work your thighs as you walk, and how to tone the upper arms at the same time.

In other words, Fitness Walking Plus is Fitness Walking plus Target Toning. You will use Target Toning exercises to address the most notorious trouble spots: the gut, the butt, the thighs, and the upper arms.

What Does Strength Training Mean to You?

Does the phrase "strength training" make you think of Arnold Schwarzenegger's bulging biceps, Olympic power lifting, or Mr. Universe wanna-bes hefting barbells in a sweaty weight room? While these are examples of extreme strength training, *ShapeWalking* takes a much simpler and friendlier approach.

ShapeWalking uses your own body weight, flexible exercise bands, and light weights to create resistance for different movements, challenging your muscles to work as they move against your own weight or the weights or bands.

ShapeWalking focuses on Strength Training for several reasons: Strong muscles work better and look better, they are more efficient, they can do more work and burn more calories, and they are tighter and more shapely. They don't blow in the breeze like laundry on a clothesline.

Strength Training works on the overload principle. When you challenge a muscle to move against resistance over and over, and do it to the point of being fatigued (but not exhausted), that muscle responds by getting stronger. *ShapeWalking* moves muscles against resistance provided by your body, small weights, or an exercise band, repeating that motion 8 to 15 times. The result is muscles that are stronger, tighter, better toned, and shapelier.

Strength Training Builds a Better Shape

Strength Training is critical to burning fat and losing weight. Muscles burn calories every minute of every day—even when you are not exercising. The more muscle you have, the more calories you burn, every minute of every hour, all day and all night.

Remember, pound for pound muscles burn significantly more calories than fat. Strength Training's ability to burn calories and tone muscles makes it an essential part of body shaping.

Strength Training Is for the Bones, Too

Strength Training tones muscle and burns fat—but did you know that it also makes your bones stronger? Part of feeling good and looking good is maintaining healthful bone density so that we can stand straight with good posture. Sometimes we think of our bones like the framework of a house—an inert structure that gives us shape. But bones are quite alive and very dynamic. They respond to activity, movement, and the contraction of the muscles around them. In other words, when you strengthen a muscle, the bones in the area also get stronger.

Strength Training is an important part of preventing or reversing loss of bone density. As we age we naturally lose some bone density. And the less dense your bones are, the more susceptible they are to fracturing or breaking. Strength Training works to maintain strong bones and promote good posture and a straight back.

Target Toning

So you have trouble spots that glare back at you from the mirror? All of us do! For most of us, the trouble spots focus on the gut, butt, thighs, and arms. The special toning exercises in the Target Toning segment build on the general Strength Training section to give you bonus shaping that attacks your trouble spots.

And Finally…Flexibility

The *ShapeWalking* program also includes a stretching or flexibility component. For your body to move freely and for each joint to move effectively, you need muscle flexibility. We are not talking about those weird body contortions you see in elite gymnastics. We're simply talking about enough flexibility to prevent injury, promote strength, and allow for good posture and proper alignment.

ShapeWalking ends each workout with a brief stretching session because that is when stretching is most effective. Warm muscles simply stretch better. Stretching is also a relaxing way to end an enjoyable workout.

So there you have them, the four basic elements of the *ShapeWalking* program: Fitness Walking, Fitness Walking Plus, Strength Training, and Target Toning. Put them together with a sound nutritional program and you have an effective program for losing weight, toning muscles, and improving body shape. The only thing you need to add is your own willingness to enjoy a better body and a healthier life.

Ready? Turn the page and let's start *ShapeWalking*.

Your Notes:

....

....

....

....

....

....

....

....

....

....

....

....

....

....

....

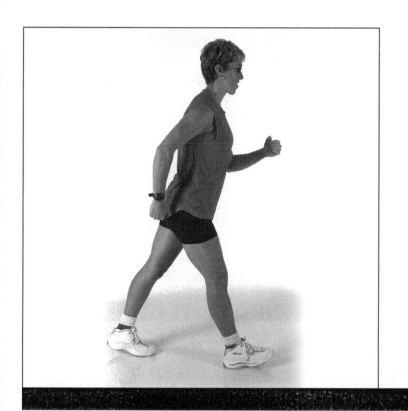

Getting Started with Fitness Walking

You have decided to learn *ShapeWalking*! Congratulations! Chapter 2 tells you everything you need to know to get started with Fitness Walking.

First Check with Your Physician

Every person over the age of twenty-five should get a physician's OK to start a walking program, especially those who do not exercise vigorously. The doctor will make sure you are good to go and can offer basic advice about where to start. If you have any nagging aches and pains in your back, legs, or shoulders, you might want to get those checked out to make sure they won't hinder your walking.

Make Sure You Have the Right Equipment

Once you get your physician's OK, you should then focus on making sure you have good walking shoes and the right clothing.

For the Love of Feet

A big part of walking is some not very fancy but very fundamental footwork. The feet work to absorb shock, helping the body land gently with each step. They also work to generate power, propelling the body forward. In fact, for every mile you walk, each foot makes thousands of shock-absorbing, body-propelling steps. In return for their hard work, the feet demand (and rightly deserve) a little bit of attention.

Taking care of your feet begins with putting them in a good pair of shoes. Go to a reputable athletic store and ask a knowledgeable salesperson for a good walking or running shoe. Shop at the end of the day when your feet are at their largest. If you wear orthotics, be sure to take them with you. Also, try on shoes while wearing the socks you will walk in. A good shoe has a top that lets the feet "breathe" while walking, allowing air to circulate and moisture to escape. Rubber and plastic don't "breathe," and rubber or plastic walking shoes will create very unhappy, sweaty feet.

Look for a cushioned, flexible sole for effective shock absorption and a heel that allows your foot to rock from heel to toe. The shoe should bend where your feet bend. When you step on it, the inside sole of the shoe should feel a little bit squishy—not like mashed potatoes, but more like a solid with a little bit of give. Check the bottom for good traction—a must, especially in wet or wintry weather.

Be sure your walking shoes respect your toes' personal space. Your toes need room to move. Look for a high and wide toe box. If you jam your foot into something too small, the toes will exact their revenge with nasty little blisters. Tingling in the toes is one sign that the shoe's toe box is too small.

The right shoe will feel good when you put it on. If it feels like it needs breaking in, put it back on the shelf—it's probably not the shoe for you. Try a different shoe or another brand. The right walking shoe should feel like slipping into something comfortable. Once you find a good brand for your feet, stick with it. Each manufacturer builds shoes around a specific foot type. The closer your foot matches the manufacturer's type, the better the fit. Try a brief little stroll down the sidewalk or around the shoe department before you purchase shoes. A little test run is the best way to decide on the right shoe.

Walking Wear

The "dress code" for walking is very loose and is not as important as having the proper shoes. Basically, suitable clothing is comfortable and allows you to move freely. At times, you might consider dressing in layers. This will allow you to adapt to changes in weather or changes in your body temperature as you get moving. As you heat up, take a layer off; if you cool down, put it back on. Reflective clothing is always a good idea for safe walking, even in the daytime.

Body clothing that wicks moisture away from your body is preferred by some walkers, but it's not as important as having wicking fabric in your socks. Your feet will also appreciate a good sock. Try athletic socks that are adequately cushioned and that have effective "wicking" properties that draw the perspiration away from your feet. Look for synthetic materials such as CoolMax, Dri-FIT, or SorbTek. If blisters are a problem, try wearing the socks inside out so the seams aren't against your skin.

Be sure your walking shoes have good traction, especially if you will be exposed

to wet or wintry weather. Also, be sure to wear sunscreen with a sun protection factor (SPF) of 15 or higher to filter out harmful ultraviolet rays. Yes, even in the winter! Cold weather actually heightens the skin's sun susceptibility.

Exercising in Hot Weather

When it's hot, fishnet or loose cotton clothing is suggested. Dress in layers so that you can remove outer clothing as you approach your target zone. Avoid restrictive clothing or materials that prevent evaporation of sweat, such as nylon.

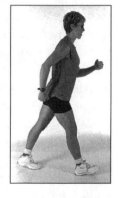

Wear a cap with a visor to protect your head from the sun and partially shade your eyes. Sunglasses will cut the sun's glare and reduce the strain on your eyes.

Take special precautions when it's hot and humid. Drink plenty of water; cut your exercise session when you become uncomfortable. Do not drink alcohol before or during your exercise session. It will dehydrate you! Begin your warm-up slowly to allow your body to adjust to the heat.

Exercising in Cold Weather

Walking in a winter wonderland can be wonderful, if you dress right. Extreme situations should always be avoided, but otherwise walking in the winter is safe.

In cold weather, 20 to 60 percent of heat is lost through an uncovered head. When the temperature dips below freezing, keep your head covered by wearing a hat. When it's too warm for a hat, a headband is a great way to keep the ears covered.

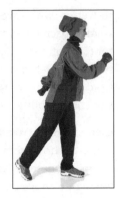

The fingers, nose, and chin get cold the most quickly, so take special care to protect them. When it is cold, wear gloves. If it is really cold, wear mittens. A scarf can be used to keep your chin and nose warm. Polar Fleece may work especially well for scarves, headbands, and mittens because it does not trap moisture. Finally, a waterproof outer shell and pants, preferably of "breathable" material, are recommended to keep the rain and snow away and the wind at bay.

The Wicking Layer—Inner

Wear nonabsorbent materials like polyester, olefin, synthetic polyester, polypropylene, or thermax for socks, hats, and underwear.

The Insulation Layer—Middle

Wear fabrics such as Thinsulate, Polar Plus, and Polar Fleece for jacket liners and pullovers.

The Protective Layer—Outer

Wear water repellent, breathable fabrics like Versatech and Gamex for light exercise. For extreme weather conditions, wear high-tech laminates that are waterproof with moderate breathability, like Gore-Tex and Thintech.

Wear shoes with adequate grip. For particularly slippery surfaces, shoe chains are available in running stores.

On cold, windy days, walk against the wind at first and return with the wind at your back. This way, perspiration will not cool on your skin and chill your body.

Start Walking

OK. Shoes on. Comfortable clothes on. Let's learn Fitness Walking!

Fitness Walking is a variation of everyday walking that provides essential aerobic activity. Fitness Walking begins with a little technique—but don't let that scare you. It's easy to learn. Fitness Walking is basically regular walking with a few minor tweaks.

Start by standing tall. Straighten your back. Hold your head high. Bring your shoulders slightly back. Now stay that way. You'll be tempted to lean forward at the waist when you get going, but stay tall. You will also be tempted to hunch your shoulders up and/or roll them forward. Keep them slightly back and relaxed.

Now hold your hands in a loose fist and bend your arms 90 degrees at the elbow. Next, pump your arms back and forth, making sure the elbows stay close to the body and the shoulders remain slightly back and relaxed. Pumping your arms back and forth puts the power in Fitness Walking. Your arms should swing in a natural arc along your body, but not cross in front of the midline of your body. Pumping the arms defines Fitness Walking more than any other motion, so work to get it right. As you tire, focus on maintaining the pumping motion of your arms. The rest of your body will just follow along.

Next, concentrate on your feet. As you bring each foot to the ground, your heel should strike first. Then, allow your foot to roll from heel to toe. Landing with a flat foot is less energy efficient and can predispose the foot to injury. If striking with your heel is difficult, try stretching your calf muscles. Tightness in this area can hinder proper Fitness Walking technique. Maintain this heel-to-toe rhythm throughout your walk.

Finish each step by pushing off from the ball of your foot (toe push-off) for a little extra power. This power push-off is accomplished by the calf muscles. It works to propel you ahead. It can also help develop some very shapely lower legs.

To get even more speed out of your Fitness Walking form, pump the arms more vigorously and shorten your stride, taking smaller, quicker steps.

Standing tall, pumping the arms, and rolling from heel to toe are the "minor tweaks" that transform regular walking

into Fitness Walking. These changes allow you to generate more power, move faster, and burn more fat and calories. Fitness Walking is like regular walking on caffeine. At its core is regular everyday walking, with a few embellishments to give it a little extra kick to really get you going.

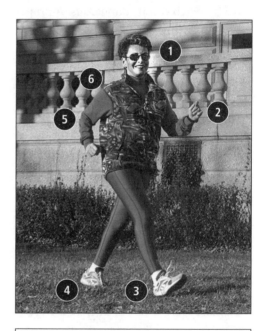

REMEMBER TO

1. Stand tall with head up
2. Keep hands in a loose fist
3. Land on your heel
4. Push with your toe
5. Bend elbows 90 degrees, keeping them close to the body and swinging
6. Keep shoulders slightly back and relaxed

Step 2: Getting Started with Fitness Walking

Warming Up, Cooling Down, and Stretching

Your muscles take some time to get loose, comfortable, and warmed up. If you jump right into fast walking, you might feel sluggish for the first few minutes. Also, jumping in too fast can raise your heart rate too quickly, which can be dangerous. A proper warm-up will gradually raise your heart rate. It provides a smooth transition from resting to moving. It prepares the body to move, so the risk of injury is lessened. To warm up for Fitness Walking, walk at a comfortable pace for a few minutes. This will get your blood moving and your heart pumping. After a few minutes, speed up to your desired walking intensity.

After walking, your body needs a little slow-down transition. When you follow the complete *ShapeWalking* program, you will also end with stretching that helps to cool you down after a workout.

Walking in the "Target Zone"

For Fitness Walking to do its fat-burning, body-shaping work, you have to walk at the right intensity. We call this the target zone. That means warming up, then walking quickly enough to reach a heart rate of 65 to 85 percent of your maximum heart rate and continuing to walk at that rate until it's time for your cooldown. Walking too slowly is not as beneficial as walking with adequate intensity. Walking too quickly can lead to fatigue.

So how do you know if you are walking at the correct speed? There are three ways to make sure you are walking in your target zone: taking the talk test, using the perceived exertion rate, and monitoring your pulse rate.

Target Zone: The Talk Test

This is the fastest and easiest way to check your effort. Just ask yourself, "Could I answer a question asked by a friend walking beside me now?" If you answer, "No, I'm too out of breath, it would be difficult or impossible to answer a question with a simple sentence without pausing for breath," slow down immediately!

If you answer, "Yes, I could say a simple sentence without pausing for breath right now. In fact, I think I could work a little harder!" try to speed up and increase your effort just a bit. Keep giving yourself the talk test, and as soon as you think you couldn't "walk the walk and talk the talk," slow down!

Target Zone: Perceived Exertion

Another way to measure the intensity of your walking session is to rate your perceived exertion. That is a fancy way to say, "keep track of how hard you feel you are working." Exercise physiologists have created a scale for this, cleverly called the "Rating of Perceived Exertion Scale" (see the scale on page 16). You can use this scale to rate how hard you're working.

The scale runs from Level 0 to 10. Level 0 is how you feel when you're sitting on the couch doing nothing. Couch potatoes live in the 0 zone. Level 10 is how you feel with extreme exertion, like when you're running through the jungle being chased by a pack of wild hyenas. Uphill. For 2 miles. Level 10 is way too hard for walking.

The walking target zone is between Levels 5 and 7. That's definitely above a "stroll in the park" but well below "this breath could be my last." Level 5 is walking deliberately, as if you are on your way to an appointment. Level 6 is walking as if you're 5 minutes late for an appointment. You're moving fast, covering ground quickly. Level 7 is walking as if you're 10 minutes late for an appointment, or as if the lottery office is closing in 3 minutes and you are still two blocks away with the million-dollar winning ticket in your hand. At Level 7 you are seriously hustling your buns, moving as efficiently as your body will smoothly allow.

Target Zone: Taking Your Pulse

The talk test and the perceived exertion scale are completely adequate for measuring the intensity of your workout. But if you want to track your intensity more closely, you can use your pulse rate for more exact levels.

This method is a little more complicated than the talk test or perceived exertion scale because you will actually take your pulse to measure the number of beats per minute. As you walk, your heart rate changes. The harder you work, the faster your heart beats. This third method uses your heart rate, as measured by your pulse beats per minute, to determine how hard you are working while you walk.

The target zone for each person is based on two factors: a scale of maximum heart rate for the person's age and the proportionate ideal heart rate for training. The ideal heart rate for working at the best intensity is 65 to 85 percent of the maximum heart rate for your age.

Don't be scared away by these concepts. The process of determining the target zone for your age, complete with age charts and examples, is described in Appendix A. But there is an "on the street," one-figure method of determining whether you are exercising at that 65 to 85 percent rate that is your target zone.

Obviously, stopping to take your pulse for a whole minute in the middle of Fitness Walking disrupts your exercise, so a shorter measurement is preferable. To use this one-figure method while exercising, slow down, look at your watch, and take your pulse for 10 seconds, counting the number of heartbeats that occur in that amount of time (you can multiply this number by six if you want to determine the number of heartbeats per minute). The one-figure method translates your 10-second pulse rate (beats per 10 seconds) into your target zone. Use the tips of your index and middle fingers to

HOW DO YOU THINK YOU FEEL?
Rating of Perceived Exertion Scale

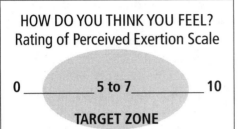

0 _____ 5 to 7 _____ 10

TARGET ZONE

LEVEL

0 = No exertion—same feeling you have when simply awake and relaxed

1 = Very slight exertion—very weak

2 = Slightly more exertion, but still weak

3 = Light to moderate exertion

4 = Moderate exertion

5 = Moderate to strong exertion— same feeling you have when walking deliberately as if on your way to an appointment

6 = Strong exertion—same feeling you have when walking as if you are 5 minutes late for an appointment

7 = Stronger exertion—same feeling you have when walking as if you are 10 minutes late for an appointment

8 = Increased exertion over Level 7— definitely exerting but you can finish your walking routine

9 = Very strong exertion, increased exertion over Level 8—you can't talk and continue walking. You should not be experiencing a Level 9 on a routine basis and should slow down or quit for the session if you feel you are working at a Level 9.

10 = Extreme exertion—same feeling you have with all-out physical activity. You should never experience a Level 10.

find your pulse at the wrist or neck. Don't use the thumb; it has a pulse of its own.

Most people find it easiest to use the "Ten-Second Target Zone" chart below for various ages. Just use the numbers for the age that is closest to your age.

For example, if you are a sassy 43-year-old on a mission to stay fit, your 10-second pulse should be between 20 and 26 for you to be working at your best intensity.

If taking your own pulse is a bit too tedious, you can wear a commercially available heart-rate monitor that will take your pulse for you. This device is strapped around your chest. It provides continuous feedback about your heart rate so you can easily determine if you are in your target zone. Sporting goods stores carry this product.

TEN-SECOND TARGET ZONE
The One-Figure Method

AGE	TEN-SECOND PULSE RATE (BEATS PER 10 SECONDS)
20	22 to 28
30	21 to 27
40	20 to 26
50	18 to 24
60	17 to 23
70	16 to 21

Hit the Road (or Sidewalk or Trail)

Now that you're dressing like a walker, walking like a walker, and finding your target zone, it's time to take yourself for a little road test. The goal is to figure out your current walking duration. We are going to find your **baseline** walking fitness level.

Start by walking for a few minutes at a comfortable pace to warm up your body so it's ready to really move. Then, look at your watch, note the time, and start walking deliberately, as though you are on your way to an appointment (Level 5 on the exertion scale). If that is too easy, walk as though you are 5 minutes late for an appointment (Level 6 on the exertion scale). If you want, you can double check to be sure you are in your target zone by taking your pulse and comparing it with the heart rate target zone. Keep walking at

this pace until you are breathing hard or with some difficulty, then slow down and check your watch again. As you cool down by walking slowly for a few minutes, figure out how long you were walking. This is your **baseline** walking fitness level, or how long you can walk in your target zone. Continue cooling down by dropping your arms from the bent position and stroll for a few minutes to gradually slow your heart rate. Your breathing should also slow down, gradually returning to normal.

Congratulations on finishing your first Fitness Walking session.

The Treadmill: A Terrific Choice for Indoor Exercise

For bad-weather days, a treadmill is a terrific choice for indoor exercise. Fitness Walking on a treadmill uses the same muscles as Fitness Walking in a mall or park—the technical differences are insignificant. Use the same technique presented above. Remember to stretch at the end of your treadmill workout.

The Next Step—Creating Your Own Walking Program

Nobody goes walking just to wear out shoes. You chose walking for a specific purpose, like getting fit, shaping up, or losing weight. To accomplish these goals, you must progress through a walking program. A walking program starts at your baseline

FINDING YOUR FITNESS WALKING BASELINE
WARM-UP
5 to 7 minutes
STARTING BASELINE
Begin – Walk at Target Zone – End*
COOL-DOWN
5 to 7 minutes
*End equals you are breathing hard or with some difficulty.

walking fitness level, then logically and safely progresses to higher levels. It is a "road map" to greater fitness.

The first element to consider in your walking program is frequency, or how often you exercise. The American College of Sports Medicine (the fitness experts) recommends moderate activity on most, if not all, days of the week, so start and maintain your program at a frequency of 5 days per week.

Next, consider duration, or how long you walk. Your baseline duration was established during the road test. If, after warming up, you walked for 10 minutes, that is your baseline duration. For the first week of your walking program, try to walk 5 days at your baseline duration.

To progress in your walking program, work on increasing the duration. Every week try to walk longer, on average, than the previous week. How much longer? Some experts recommend the 10 percent rule—walking an average of 10 percent longer each week. As long as the average walk duration each week is longer than it was the week before, your walking program is on target. You will likely have some days of the week where you have more time (or energy) than others. It is fine to vary the duration of walks on different days; just be sure the average length is increasing. For example, if you are shooting to average 14 minutes per day, walking as far as 16 minutes or as little as 12 minutes is OK. Also, dramatic differences in walking length are not recommended in the early stages of a Fitness Walking program.

MODEL PROGRESSION CHART

WEEK	DURATION	FREQUENCY	INTENSITY LEVEL
1	10 minutes	5 times/week	5–6
2	11.5 minutes	5 times/week	5–6
3	13 minutes	5 times/week	5–6
4	14.5 minutes	5 times/week	5–6
5	16 minutes	5 times/week	5–6
6	18 minutes	5 times/week	5–6
7	18 minutes	5 times/week	5–7
8	20 minutes	5 times/week	5–7
9	22.5 minutes	5 times/week	5–7
10	25 minutes	5 times/week	5–7

NOTE: All bold figures indicate an increase in duration or intensity.

Sharon, for example, walked for 12 minutes each outing during the first week of her walking program. Some days she felt like she could do more, but she stuck with the 12 minutes to be certain not to overdo it. The second week she increased her average walk to 14 minutes, a reasonable next step in her walking program. During this second week, she walked for 14 minutes 3 times. One day she was short on time and only squeezed in a 12-minute walk. Her fifth walk was 16-minutes long. Although these walks were of varying lengths, the average was 14 minutes.

As you become a seasoned walker, you can vary walking duration more because your body will be used to longer walks. Just be sure you do not make dramatic increases in the duration of your longest walk. If your longest walk has been 30 minutes, do not suddenly go up to 45 minutes. Work your way up gradually.

The Ups and Downs of Hill Walking

Whether the road rises up or slopes down before you, maintain your tall, upright walking form. You will be inclined to bend forward and lean into it as you walk uphill. Instead stand tall and shorten your stride slightly.

Walking downhill can also challenge your posture. Keep your body straight, allowing gravity to help pull you down the hill, but keep it smooth. Maintain the heel-to-toe motion of your feet. If you're landing with a jarring motion, slow down. Keep your stride smooth and controlled.

Stretching

Stretching is an important part of basic body maintenance. When you use your muscles, they contract or shorten. If you do not incorporate stretching into your fitness routine, your muscles can get chronically shortened. This leads to muscle imbalances that may cause injuries. Muscle imbalances can also cause poor posture—and there is nothing flattering about the hunched-over Cro-Magnon look.

The *ShapeWalking* stretching program consists of four simple stretches. Each stretch is designed to address a flexibility "hot spot"—an area particularly prone to loss of range of motion. Do this stretching after you finish your workout for the day, regardless of which parts of the program you do: Fitness Walking, Fitness Walking Plus, Strength Training, or Target Toning. It will be 2 minutes and 40 seconds well spent.

Pectoral Stretch

Stand tall with your abdominals in and your knees and shoulders relaxed.

Place your arms, elbows bent, in front of your body just below shoulder level. Turn your hands so that your palms face outward (the backs of your hands face your body). Pull your shoulder blades down and together in one motion while bringing your elbows back. Feel a gentle stretch along the front of the shoulders. Initially, hold for 10 seconds; release and stretch more deeply for 30 seconds.

Calf Stretch

Stand with your hands on a sturdy surface. Place one foot behind you, with your toes pointing forward. While keeping your body straight and your heels on the floor, lean forward to feel a gentle stretch in the calf of the back leg. Initially, hold for 10 seconds; release and stretch more deeply for 30 seconds. Repeat on the opposite side.

Thigh and Hip Stretch

Standing upright with your hands on a sturdy surface, bring one heel to your but-

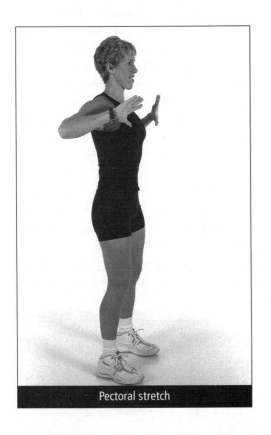

Pectoral stretch

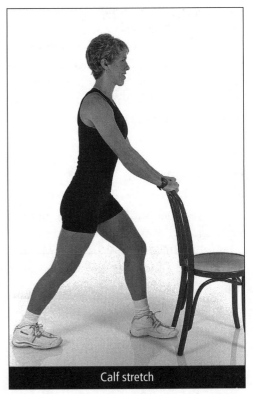

Calf stretch

tocks by grasping the foot with your hand. Do not lean forward at the waist. Feel a gentle stretch along the front of the thigh and hip. Initially, hold for 10 seconds; release and stretch more deeply for 30 seconds. Repeat on the opposite side.

Hamstring Stretch

Stand with your lower back straight and one foot elevated about 1 to 2 feet (on a step, park bench, chair). Then lean forward from the hip. Do not round your back. Feel a gentle stretch along the back of the thigh. Initially, hold for 10 seconds;

release and stretch more deeply for 30 seconds. Repeat on the opposite side.

Other Important Stuff

You now have the tools you need to start your Fitness Walking program, but there are a few other issues related to your health and safety that remain to be addressed.

Keep Yourself Hydrated

According to the American College of Sports and Medicine, adequate fluid

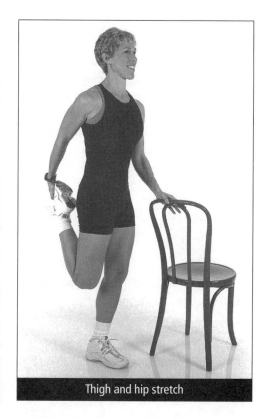
Thigh and hip stretch

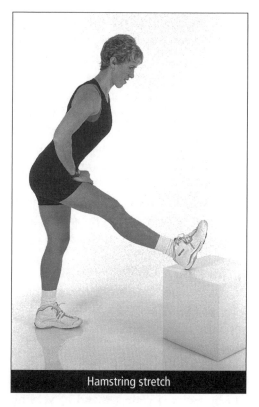
Hamstring stretch

replacement promotes health, safety, and optimizes exercise performance. Drink at least 8 cups of decaffeinated fluids per day and more when exercising. Drink 2 cups of water about 2 hours before walking.

During your walk try to drink at regular intervals in an attempt to replace the fluids lost through sweating. After your walk drink 1 to 2 cups of water to replenish fluid levels. Keep the water cooler than the ambient temperature in order to enhance absorption.

Follow Some Essential Safety Guidelines

When *ShapeWalking* outside, be alert to your surroundings. Choose paths with firm footing so you won't misstep or turn an ankle. Choose routes that are safe and well lit.

Reflective clothing, available in most athletic stores, is a safety plus. Reflective clothing is especially important for evening walks and is even a good idea for the daytime.

Carry an ID. Also, carry a cell phone or enough money for a phone call. Vary your route and stay alert. Consider inviting a friend to accompany you on your Fitness Walks.

Leave your hand weights at home! They will put you at risk for forearm and shoulder injuries and can increase your blood pressure.

So there it is—everything you need to start your walking program. You can add fun by walking with a friend or varying your route. But the most fun of all will come from walking longer, feeling better, and becoming more fit.

The Goal

The long-term goal is to walk for 45 to 60 minutes 3 times per week, and about 30 minutes 2 times per week. Again, an important word of caution: increase your walking duration gradually. Most people who quit a new fitness program do so because of soreness or injury sustained from going too hard or too fast. Protect yourself from injury. Start gradually and stick with it for the long haul.

Below is a brief review of the important elements in your walking program. When you are ready to plan a weekly Fitnes Walking program, refer to the blank "Fitness Walking Record" on page 116. This worksheet will help you organize your goals for the weeks ahead.

WALKING PROGRAM
HOW OFTEN?
5 times per week.
HOW HARD?
Work in your target zone (either heart-rate zone or perceived exertion zone).
HOW LONG?
Start with your baseline duration and gradually work up to 45 to 60 minutes 3 times per week, and 30 minutes 2 times per week.

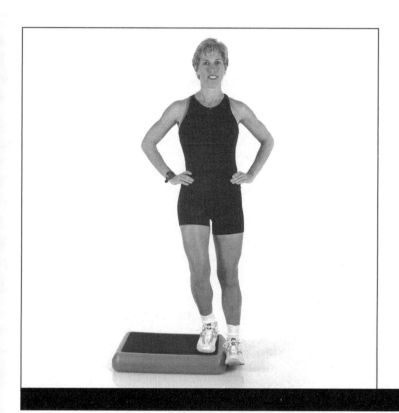

Fitness Walking Plus

If you want to "kick-up" your walking outing to burn extra calories and firm your abs, buttocks, and thighs—all in a single workout—then Fitness Walking Plus is for you. Fitness Walking Plus adds bonus shaping exercises to Fitness Walking to firm these trouble spots—all during your walking outing.

Step 3: Fitness Walking Plus

Add the Plus to Fitness Walking

Fitness Walking is a great way to get fit. Fitness Walking Plus is a great way to get fit and specifically shape your body. Fitness Walking Plus is Fitness Walking enhanced by toning exercises for the abs, butt, thighs, and upper arms that are to be performed during your walk. It's like taking a very nice, functional wardrobe and adding some splashy color and clever accessories. Or turning your minivan into a sleek convertible. Fitness Walking Plus allows you to go beyond the benefits of Fitness Walking and add some shaping to your body's trouble spots.

Fitness Walking is an aerobic activity. It works to improve your heart's health, burn calories and fat, and help you become slimmer. Fitness Walking will help you lose weight, but by itself it is not enough exercise if you want to achieve an ideal body shape.

The Plus in Fitness Walking Plus is the addition of some simple muscle-toning exercises. You can put the Plus in Fitness Walking by tightening specific muscles such as the abdominals as you are walking, causing them to work harder and get stronger. Or you can add specific non-walking movements to strengthen targeted muscles such as the triceps. These two toning strategies will strengthen muscles during your outing, toning muscles as you burn fat.

Fitness Walking Plus works particular muscle groups to help you look and function your best. Fitness Walking Plus provides extra emphasis on selected areas, but it does not replace your overall conditioning program. In fact, you will not get your best results without an overall conditioning program, so be sure to do your *ShapeWalking* Strength Training program at least 2, preferably 3, times per week (see Step 4 starting on page 35).

At the top of the body-shaping "most-wanted" list are the abs, butt, thighs, and upper arms. These are the areas most people want to shape up. What puts the jiggle and wiggle in these trouble spots? The answer is fat.

Fat is a subcutaneous tissue, which means it sits right below the skin and on top of the muscle. As we gain weight, the amount of fat throughout the body increases. But most of us also have a special little storage area where fat really wants to hang out. For example, Peter and Deb are a married couple who each gained about 10 pounds in their first year of marriage. Peter's 10 pounds found a home around his abdomen, while Deb's 10 pounds went straight to her hips.

The first route to getting rid of body fat is to lose weight. Fitness Walking will do that for you, and Strength Training (which we will cover later) will help as well. Fitness Walking Plus adds a strengthening component to Fitness Walking for further ammunition in eliminating those troublesome fat strongholds. Add a sensible diet to the mix and you will be on your way to achieving a better body.

That Sassy Cellulite

First, a word about that doughy, dimply doggone tenacious tissue called cellulite. Cellulite looks a little different, but it's really just fat. It gets its dimply appearance because of the way it is attached to the muscle underneath it, but it's still just fat. The thighs and buttocks are cellulite's favorite hangouts. To get rid of cellulite, first get rid of the fat and then tone the muscles underneath. Fitness Walking Plus does double damage to cellulite. Fitness Walking burns the fat *while* the shaping strategies tone the muscles.

Toning Muscle

Shaping up isn't just about losing fat. Sometimes it's also about toning muscle. For example, if your buttocks are as flat as the plains of Nebraska, you might want to add a little sculpted, perky muscle shape to that area. Muscles give your body shape. Consequently, toning your muscles is a big part of changing and improving your body shape. Without the right toning exercises, muscles become soft and flabby. However, with toning exercises, muscles become strong and tight, creating smooth lines and sculpted curves that give your body shape.

Fitness Walking Plus is designed to tone, and thus shape up, the muscles in four specific areas: the abdomen (abs), the buttocks, the thighs, and the upper arms. You can choose which areas to work on, if any. Fitness Walking Plus challenges these muscles to work harder by tightening them as you walk (abs and buttocks), by adding a simple toning maneuver (thighs), or by adding resistance (upper arms). Remember, muscle tone can also be further enhanced in these areas (and others) through Strength Training, which we will cover in the next step (starting on page 35).

Toning Your Abs While You Walk

Somewhere under that extra skin and fat stored around your middle is a group of four muscles called the abdominal muscles. The abdominal muscles include

- **the rectus abdominus,** which runs up and down the anterior (front) surface of the trunk from the middle of the rib cage (fifth and sixth ribs near the sternum), between the rib cage and the pelvis

- **the transverse abdominus,** the deepest abdominal muscle, which starts at the middle of the rib cage (fifth and sixth ribs) and runs horizontally around the torso from the middle of the ribs to the pelvis

Step 3: Fitness Walking Plus

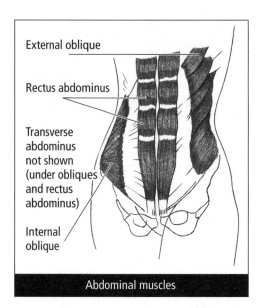

- External oblique
- Rectus abdominus
- Transverse abdominus not shown (under obliques and rectus abdominus)
- Internal oblique

Abdominal muscles

- **the external oblique**, which runs diagonally from your ribs to your hips (imagine fibers running diagonally into the front pockets of your slacks)

- **the internal oblique,** which runs along the front and sides of your torso (imagine fibers running diagonally into your back pockets). Think of the oblique muscles as your waist muscles.

These muscles hold the abdominal organs in place, support the lower back, flex the trunk, maintain an erect posture, and play an important stabilizing role in almost any activity the body undertakes. Besides that, they look really, really good when they are tight and toned.

How to Add Ab Toning to Your Fitness Walking Program

If your abdomen is one of your shaping trouble spots, first you need to get acquainted with your abdominal muscles; you need to know what it feels like when they contract or tighten. To find your abdominal muscles, stand tall with your hands along each side of your trunk just above the waist, with thumbs at the love handles and fingers pointing toward each other.

Now, tighten your stomach muscles, picturing the muscles tightening and drawing in toward your belly button. Your fingers should feel the muscles tighten.

If you try this and your ab muscles are still AWOL (absent without leave)—if you can't feel them contract or feel them tighten under your fingers—try this method: Stand with your back against the wall. Place your fingers as instructed above. Now tighten your stomach muscle, picturing the muscles tightening, and flat-

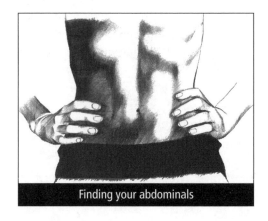

Finding your abdominals

ten your back against the wall. Your fingers should feel the muscles contract. Practice this until you have a good feel for what it is like when your stomach muscles tighten.

Next, stand tall (without your back against the wall) and tighten your stomach muscles without relying on your fingers to feel the contraction. As this gets easier, tighten your stomach muscles while walking around. When you can reliably feel them tightening, you are ready to tone your abdominal muscles while you walk.

After warming up with moderate-paced walking, start your Fitness Walking at a quicker pace, maintaining proper form. Now, hold your abdominal muscles tight, sucking them into your belly button while you walk. Do not let this interfere with your breathing. Your breathing should remain steady. Also, remind yourself not to bend forward at the waist as you tighten the stomach muscles. Maintain your tall and straight walking posture. Hold this muscle contraction for a count of 4, then release. Gradually build up to be able to hold the contraction for a count of 10, always remembering to breathe naturally. Then, give yourself a 2-minute rest and contract them again. Remind yourself frequently to retighten your abdominal muscles throughout your walk, as the tight contraction may slowly fade as you get tired. Repeat this routine as follows:

1. tighten your muscles until they fatigue

2. take a 2-minute rest

3. retighten your muscles

4. take a 2-minute rest

Over time, you should be able to hold the contraction longer and longer. In fact, some walkers hold a conscious stomach-muscle contraction for a whole 45-minute walk. Those are some rock-hard abdominal muscles!

A Bit About the Butt

Shaping problems related to the butt are usually one of two extremes: either too much or too little. Let's start with the too much end of things. First, you must determine what you have too much of by doing the pinch test. While standing, pinch your butt (middle of the cheek) with your thumb and forefinger. If it pinches, it's fat. If it doesn't pinch, it's muscle. If your butt is all muscle, you don't need more shaping or conditioning for the butt muscles. In fact, you should avoid doing any strength training for these muscles so you don't increase muscle mass. Concentrate on Fitness Walking and on Strength Training for other areas.

Fitness Walking Plus is the answer both for too much fat in the butt and for

Step 3: Fitness Walking Plus

too little tone, because the walking component burns up the fat while the toning
component tones the muscles. If too much
fat is your trouble, emphasize Fitness
Walking to burn extra calories, but be sure
to also tone your derrière by incorporating
Fitness Walking Plus's butt-toning moves.
If too little tone is your buttocks issue, focus
on the butt-toning component in Fitness
Walking Plus and consider using Fitness
Walking Plus buttocks toning every
minute of every walk you take. It will take
some time to work up to that goal, but
your butt muscles should respond with better tone and greater shape.

If your butt is abundant with fat, work
to tone your derrière and to burn fat. The
main muscle in the buttocks is the gluteus
maximus. The gluteus maximus and the

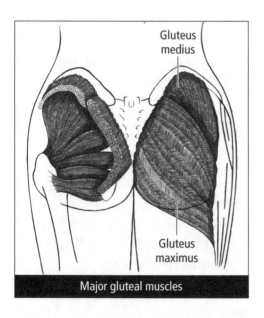

Major gluteal muscles

Gluteus
medius

Gluteus
maximus

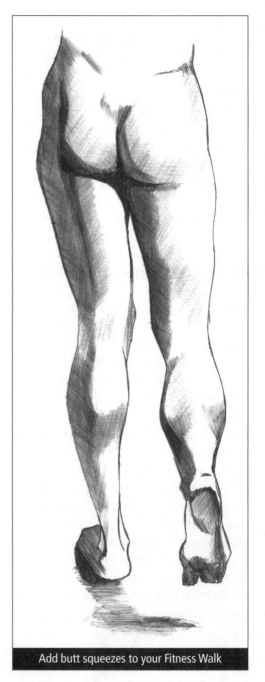

Add butt squeezes to your Fitness Walk

other butt muscles work to extend the hip. In other words, whenever the foot is on the ground, this muscle works to power the body forward. You can shape these butt muscles by tightening them when the foot is on the ground while you walk. Let's learn how that is done.

Toning Your Butt

First, get acquainted with your butt muscles so you will know how to tighten or contract them. Try squeezing your butt cheeks while standing still. You can use your hands to feel the muscles tighten. Think of pulling each cheek forward and up (closer to your body). When you can do this, try walking slowly and squeezing the butt cheek of the leg that is on the ground. Start squeezing just after the heel strike and continue squeezing until just before the toe pushes off. Remember, the foot touching the ground has the butt cheek tightened.

This process takes practice. When you can do this, you are ready for Fitness Walking Plus shaping for the buttocks.

Begin your Fitness Walking workout. When you're moving well, tighten the butt muscles of the leg that is on the ground right after the heel strike and into the push-off. When you pick up the foot, relax the muscles. As you walk, you will alternately tighten one butt cheek, then the other as you place one foot, then the other on the ground. You will feel the contraction best right before your heel comes off

the ground, and you can emphasize the tightening at this point.

Initially, shaping the butt while Fitness Walking might require a bit of concentration, but later it will become second nature. The pay-off—a tight, toned butt—will be worth the effort. Gradually add butt-shaping to your Fitness Walking outings. Initially, add butt-shaping moves for 1 minute, then resume Fitness Walking for 2 minutes. Build up to adding butt squeezes for longer periods of time during your walk.

The Thighs Have It

Saddlebags and saggy knees—so go the body-shaping woes of the thighs. The source of these trouble spots is typically stored fat (saddlebags) and unconditioned muscle (saggy knees). Fitness Walking Plus has a simple strategy to strengthen the thigh muscles and eliminate unwanted fat.

The hip abductors and lateral quadriceps muscles run along the outside of the hip and thigh. These muscles stabilize the hip and pelvis laterally (sideways) during walking and support proper knee function. The quadriceps muscles run along the front of the thigh, and they support the knee and absorb shock as you walk.

Saddlebags are the result of stored fat along the outside of the hip and thigh. Some people, especially women, are particularly prone to this thigh-toning problem. Every ounce of weight they gain

Step 3: Fitness Walking Plus

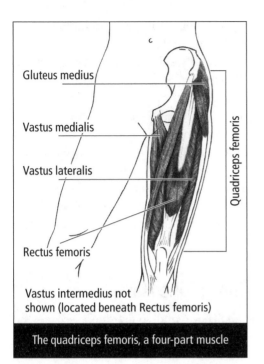

Gluteus medius

Vastus medialis

Vastus lateralis

Quadriceps femoris

Rectus femoris

Vastus intermedius not shown (located beneath Rectus femoris)

The quadriceps femoris, a four-part muscle

seems to go straight to this area. Fitness Walking Plus thigh toning delivers a double whammy to the saddlebags. Fitness Walking burns up the stored fat, while the toning part tones the lateral thigh and hip muscles.

When they are not properly toned, the front of the thighs can look saggy and flabby. Saggy knees develop from unconditioned quadriceps muscles along the front of the thigh. When properly toned, these muscles create shapely thighs, decimating saggy knees.

Toning Your Thighs

Fitness Walking Plus has three simple methods for eliminating thigh problems by toning: side step down, hill walking, and stair climbing. Side step down works both the hip abductor muscles along the outside of the hip and the quadriceps muscles along the front and outside of the thigh. Hill walking and stair climbing both work the quadriceps muscles on the front of the thigh.

Side Step Down

The first thigh-toning maneuver, the one that works both the side and the front muscles, is called a side step down. It requires a curb or step that you can move up and down on sideways. If you choose a curb, for your safety stay away from traffic and be alert for cars. Or find a step along your path, perhaps leading into a yard or park.

Stand on one foot at the edge of the step or curb with your body parallel to the step or curb. Now, bend the knee of the leg that is up on the step, slowly lower the opposite foot to the street or sidewalk below, and lightly touch down with the heel of the lower foot.

Be certain to keep your hips level during this exercise—you will be tempted to let the hip drop on the side you are lowering down. Also, the foot that you are lowering should stay parallel to the ground

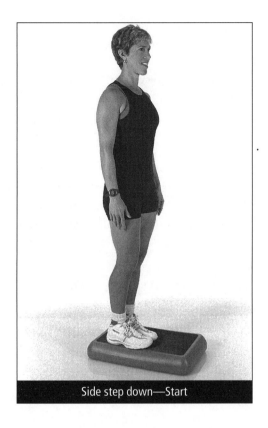

Side step down—Start

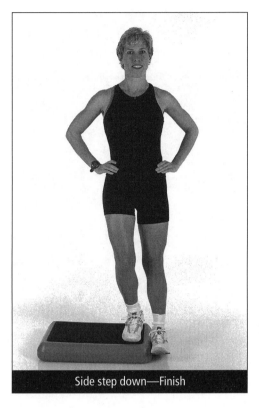

Side step down—Finish

and should just touch down lightly at the heel. Do not push off with this foot. This exercise works the front and outside muscles of the leg you're standing on, and proper technique will let these muscles do the work.

Begin with 10 repetitions of this exercise on each side. Gradually, work up to 2 or 3 sets, sprinkling them throughout your walk. For example, you might walk 10 minutes, perform 1 set of 10 repetitions, walk 10 minutes, perform a second set of 10 repetitions, and so on.

Hill Walking and Stair Climbing

Another way to work the quadriceps muscles along the front of the thigh is to walk repeatedly up either a steep hill or a flight of stairs. Choose a walking route with a steep hill at least 5 to 10 minutes into your walk. (If the hill comes too soon, you might not be sufficiently warmed up to tackle this challenge.) As you begin to climb the hill, shorten your stride and quicken your step. Emphasize the quadriceps by tightening the muscles along the front of your thigh when that foot is on the

Step 3: Fitness Walking Plus

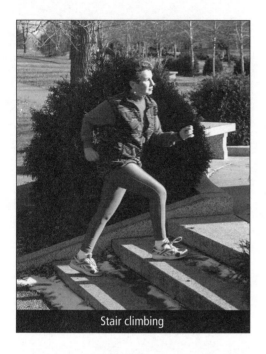

Stair climbing

ground. The quadriceps muscles should "drive" you up the hill. If the hill is short, you can walk back down and repeat the hill climb until the quads have had their workout. Or if the hill is long, continue your walk and come back to the hill later to climb it again.

Alternatively, if you pass a long flight of stairs on your walk, you can use it for a thigh-shaping challenge. As you climb the stairs, use your quadriceps muscles to "drive" you up the steps. Tighten this muscle group along the front of your thigh as you straighten the leg while moving from step to step.

You can climb a flight of stairs repeatedly if you are able, or catch it on the way out and again on the way back. If you stair

climb or hill walk for more than 2 minutes, you will also gain the benefit of an enhanced aerobic workout.

Side step downs, hill walking, and stair climbing are the Fitness Walking Plus strategies for toning your fat, flabby thighs. Use them while you Fitness Walk to tone your thighs into shape.

For effective toning, continuously challenge these muscle groups. For side step downs, search out a high step; for hill walking, find a steeper hill; for stair climbing, try a higher step or more repetitions.

The Upper-Arm Answer

The triceps muscle runs along the back of the upper arm. When these muscles are

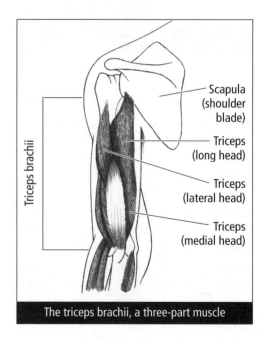

The triceps brachii, a three-part muscle

deconditioned, the arms look flabby. When toned, the arms look sleek, strong, and solid.

You can get significant upper-arm shaping by specifically adding an exercise to tone your triceps. You can do this exercise anytime you are waiting to cross the street or when you want to stop to take a break from your walk. To tone the triceps, find a piece of rubber tubing or a resistance band to take with you on your walk. (See "Starting Equipment" on page 38 for sources.) Exercise bands and tubing can be of variable resistance; some are taut and

work your muscles strenuously, while others are less taut and provide less challenge to the muscles. For this Fitness Walking Plus upper-arm–toning strategy, start with a band or tubing with minimal resistance.

While waiting at the crosswalk for the light to change, tie the band around your waist and grasp the end of the band with palms facing the body. Bring the elbow slightly behind the body and hold it stationary. Extend the forearm back, bringing it in line with the elbows.

Do 10 repetitions, gradually building up to 2 or 3 sets of 10 repetitions at a time

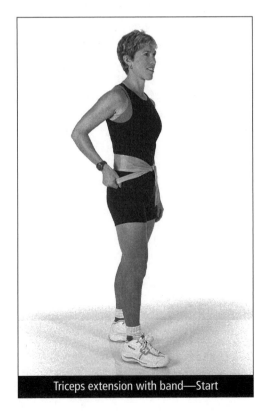

Triceps extension with band—Start

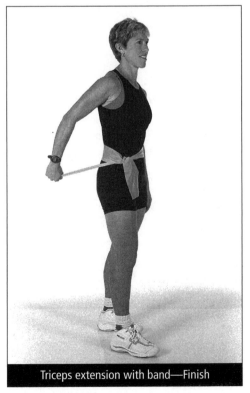

Triceps extension with band—Finish

intermittently during your walk. Try eventually to fit in 2 or 3 arm-shaping sessions during your walk. When comfortable, try exercising both arms at the same time. When stopping to perform your arm shaping, march in place to keep your heart rate elevated. To effectively tone these muscles, gradually increase the resistance of the band.

If you experience any pain in the shoulders while doing Fitness Walking Plus upper-arm shaping, stop using the band and continue with your normal fitness walk. The next time out, try a band with less resistance. If you still experience pain, this toning exercise is not for you.

Stretching

Fitness Walking Plus will tone your muscles. But remember to keep them limber with stretching as well. Every time you conclude your *ShapeWalking* activities, whether basic *Fitness Walking* or *Fitness Walking Plus*, finish with the four simple stretches described at the end of Step 2 on pages 20–21. The 2 minutes and 40 seconds required to complete these stretches will make a tremendous difference for your muscles. Be sure to do all four stretches: pectoral, calf, thigh and hip, and hamstring. Your muscles will love you for those few minutes.

The Fitness Walking Plus Program

The four toning exercises for the abs, butt, thighs, and upper arms make up Fitness Walking Plus and can be used however you choose. Pick the ones that will help you get the body you want. You can do more than one toning exercise on any given walk. In fact, you can do them all on any given walk or do a different one every day of the week. Adding these toning exercises—putting the Plus in Fitness Walking Plus—results in a powerful weight-reducing, muscle-toning, body-shaping combination.

To help you formulate your Fitness Walking Plus program, make copies of and use the blank "Fitness Walking Plus Progression Chart" that can be found on page 117. This worksheet will help you organize your exercise plan for the weeks ahead.

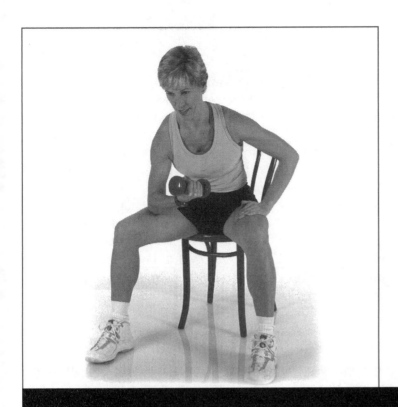

Strength Training

Fitness Walking and Fitness Walking Plus will give you all the cardiovascular work you need plus some bonus toning for your trouble spots. But a complete fitness program requires that you build muscle. The *ShapeWalking* Strength Training program is a full body-toning program that works your body's major muscle groups.

Step 4: Strength Training

Fitness Walking and Fitness Walking Plus are dynamic and effective ways to start working on looking and feeling your best. In fact, like eggs in an omelette, Fitness Walking is the main ingredient in *Shape-Walking*. Still, eggs alone don't make an omelette, and Fitness Walking alone does not make *ShapeWalking*. For optimal body shaping, you also have to add some Strength Training to your regimen. The *ShapeWalking* Strength Training program is an overall toning program that works your body's major muscle groups.

even just gravity. Muscles respond to this kind of work by getting stronger and more toned.

The *ShapeWalking* Strength Training program works the major muscle groups in the body. It is a great overall toning program. This program should be done 2 to 3 times per week, but not on consecutive days. Your body needs a day off between sessions to recover properly. Some exercises have both a beginning and an advanced level—choose the one that works best for you.

Why Strength Train?

The *ShapeWalking* Strength Training program is not about body building. Our goal is muscle strengthening/toning. Toning creates firm muscles, and firm muscles lead to a better body shape. Toned muscles are metabolically active efficient fat and calorie burners. Fat tissue, by contrast, is relatively inert. Muscle is a furnace that burns up fat, and the more muscle tone you have, the more fat you will burn. As a bonus, Strength Training also builds stronger bones that are essential for good posture. Right from the start, lay aside any ideas about hulking, bulgy muscles.

Muscles get tighter and more toned when they are challenged to work harder than they normally do. Your muscles work when they are repeatedly moving against some type of resistance: an exercise band, an ankle weight, a handheld weight, or

Just Do It Right

Before you jump into any Strength Training exercises, start with an easy warm-up to prepare the muscles for work. A warm-up will decrease the chance of injury. It will also chase the sluggishness out of your system. Any smooth, rhythmic activity that gets your heart pumping a little harder will work for a warm-up. A walk will suffice. Walking or jogging in place will also do. Or, Strength Train *after* you Fitness Walk—your muscles will definitely be warmed up then.

Perform each strengthening exercise slowly and smoothly. Maintain good posture and alignment throughout the exercise. As you tire, it will be especially tempting to lose form. Work to keep your posture as good on the tenth repetition as it was on the first.

Breathe naturally as you Strength Train. Never, ever hold your breath. Holding your breath can dangerously elevate your blood pressure. Remind yourself frequently to keep breathing normally.

Finding Your Starting Level and Progressing

Just as when you started Fitness Walking, you need to find your starting level for resistance Strength Training. First, perform the exercise without resistance and check your form. Then, try it with resistance (weights and bands are discussed in the next section) for 8 repetitions without a rest. (A rep is defined as the single and complete action of the exercise from start to finish and back to the starting position.) The last repetition should be difficult to complete, and you should experience some muscle fatigue. If you can't do all 8 repetitions, do as many as you can. That is your starting point. If you can easily do 8 repetitions, try 10. If you can easily do 10 reps, try 12. If you can easily do 12 reps, go to the next higher resistance or weight level. Repeat this process until you find your starting level and starting number of repetitions. Remember, for different exercises you may have different starting levels. As you get stronger, progress gradually as is comfortable for your body.

For each exercise, count to 2 for each phase of the movement: lifting, holding, and returning. For example, lift for 2 counts, hold for 2 counts, and take 2 counts to return to the starting position. As you progress, count to 4 for each phase of the exercise: Lift for 4 counts, hold for 4 counts, and return to the starting position for 4 counts.

For exercises that use only your body weight (no resistance bands or weights), start with 8 repetitions or do as many as you can. Progress by moving to 10 and then 12 repetitions. To further progress, complete the advanced versions of the exercises presented in the latter part of this chapter. For example, progress from the beginner's heel raise-toe raise to the advanced heel raise-toe raise.

Every time you perform a resistance strength exercise, it counts as a *rep* (short for repetition). In order to build muscle, it's not enough to do 1 repetition per exercise, because the muscle you are strengthening needs to be challenged repeatedly. For every exercise in this chapter, you should perform 8 to 12 reps in a row without interruption.

A *set* consists of a given number of complete and continuous reps of a single exercise. A set in this Strength Training program is 8 to 12 repetitions of the same exercise.

If, after a complete workout, you find that doing 1 set per exercise is too easy, you can either repeat the strength-training exercises, increase the number of reps per set, or do 2 sets per exercise the next time around. If your schedule and level of vigor

Step 4: Strength Training

permit, do 1 to 3 sets of any exercise that is important to your goals. Make sure you increase the number of reps or sets gradually to prevent injury and/or exhaustion. If you haven't worked out for a long time, it's always recommended that you start off easily and then slowly increase your workload.

The latter part of this chapter presents explanations of each Strength Training resistance exercise's start and end position, accompanied by photographs to help you complete each exercise correctly.

To summarize, your Strength Training workouts should follow the guidelines listed below:

Frequency: 2 to 3 times each week, but not 2 days in a row

Start with: the beginner-level exercise

With the goal of: advancing in level and weight, as much as you are able

Reps: 8 to 12 per set

Sets: at least 1 set per exercise, preferably 2 sets per exercise

Count: start with 2 counts for each phase; progress to 4 counts for each phase

---

Starting Equipment

This Strength Training program requires minimal equipment. To get started, a set of ankle weights, two small hand weights, and one medium hand weight will do. As you get stronger, you may need heavier weights. Small weights are readily available in sporting goods and discount stores. To begin, you will need the following:

Dumbbells: 3-pound, 5-pound, and 8-pound dumbbells

Ankle weights: 2-pound and 5-pound ankle weights

Bands: Light-resistance pack or single band. These are available from OPTP, at (800) 367-7393, and SPRI, at (800) 222-7774.

Begin with the lightest weights and the number of repetitions best for you. If the exercises are too easy, add more weight until you find the best size weights to use for your level. As you build muscle, gradually increase the weight you use.

The *ShapeWalking* Strength Training Programs

So here it is—a simple Strength Training program that effectively tones the most important muscles. A word of caution—if any exercise causes pain in a joint, stop doing it. Some muscle soreness the day after strength training is normal, and you should expect this. Sharp pain or burning irritation in the joints is not expected, however. Skip any exercise that causes that kind of symptom in any joint.

Most of us start a new exercise program with zeal. Don't let this zealous energy cause you to do too much too fast. The number-one reason people drop out of a fitness program prematurely is because they start furiously and then get too sore to continue. Go slowly. Build up gradually. Commit to doing this right and staying with it for the long haul.

The basic program is the 30-Minute Strength Training Program, but if you are pressed for time, you can complete a 15-Minute Strength Training Program by completing only the starred exercises. For easy reference, this abbreviated program is described on page 59. As with the other components of the *ShapeWalking* program, there is a blank worksheet on page 118 that will help you organize your Strength Training program for the weeks ahead.

THE 30-MINUTE STRENGTH TRAINING PROGRAM

Heel Raise—Toe Raise

The heel raise-toe raise builds muscle in the calf (back of the lower leg) and strengthens the front of the lower leg.

Beginner Heel Raise—Toe Raise

- For balance, place your hands on the back of a sturdy chair or other firm surface.

- Lift both heels slowly off the floor, hold, and slowly lower them. Pause briefly.

- Raise the toes of both feet off the floor, hold, and slowly lower the toes to the floor. Pause.

- You will feel the heel raise in the back of your lower leg. The toe raise is felt in front of your lower leg.

- Alternate heel raises and toe raises until you have done 8 to 12 of each (16 to 24 movements).

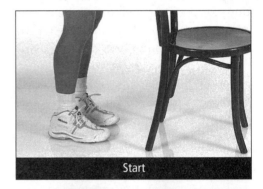
Start

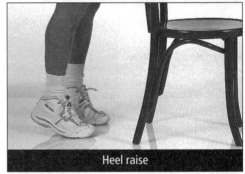
Heel raise

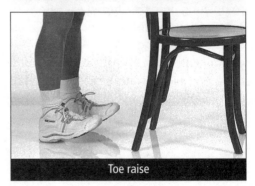
Toe raise

Advanced Heel Raise—Toe Raise

- For balance, place your hands on the back of a sturdy chair or other firm object.

- Stand on one leg. Keep posture erect.

- Lift the heel of the leg you are standing on from the floor slowly, hold, and slowly lower it. Pause briefly.

- Lift the toes of the leg you are standing on slowly, hold, and slowly lower the toes to the floor. Pause.

- Alternate heel and toe raises on one foot.

- You will feel the heel raise in the back of your lower leg; the toe raise is felt in the front of the lower leg.

- Complete 8 to 12 reps (16 to 24 movements); then repeat on the other side.

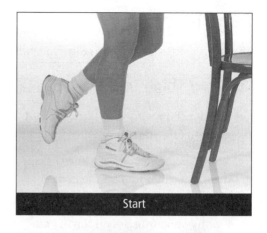

Start

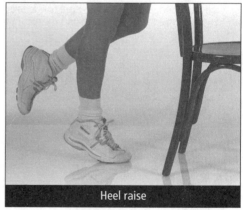

Heel raise

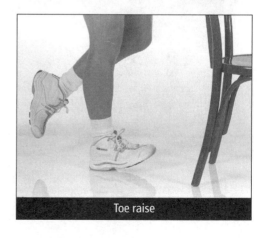

Toe raise

Thigh Toner

The thigh toner tones and firms the thigh muscles.

Beginner Thigh Toner**

- Sit on a chair with your back straight and tall and your ab muscles tight.

- While keeping your right knee bent, raise your right foot off the floor.

- Slowly straighten your leg by tightening the quad muscles on top of your thigh, hold, and slowly bend the knee.

- You will feel the work above your knee on the front of your thigh.

- Complete 8 to 12 reps, then repeat on the other leg.

- Add ankle weights as you're able.

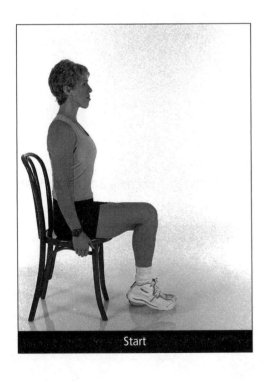

Start

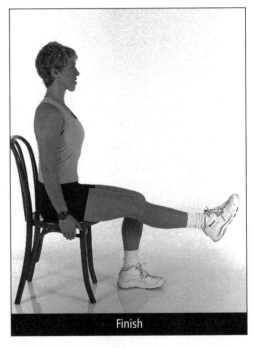

Finish

Advanced Thigh Toner**

- For balance, stand with one hand on the back of a sturdy chair or other firm surface.

- Bring your right knee up to hip level.

- Slowly straighten your leg by tightening the quad muscles on top of your thigh, hold, then slowly bend the knee.

- You will feel the work above your knee on the front of your thigh.

- Complete 8 to 12 reps, then repeat on the other leg.

- Add ankle weights as you're able.

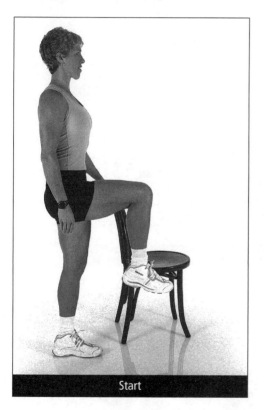

Start

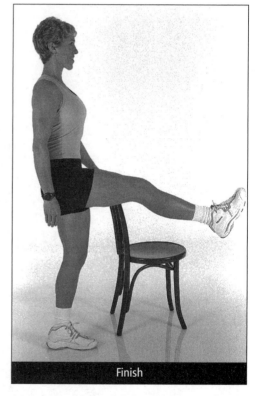

Finish

Step 4: Strength Training

Outer-Thigh and Hip Toner

The outer-thigh and hip toner firms and builds outer-thigh and hip muscles.

Beginner Outer-Thigh and Hip Toner**

- Lie on your left side with your head, shoulder, and hip aligned.

- For balance, put your right hand, palm side down, in front of you.

- Lift your right leg slowly, hold, and slowly lower it.

- You will feel the work on the outside surface of your thigh, along the side of your leg and just below your butt.

- Complete 8 to 12 reps, then repeat on the other side.

- Add ankle weights as you're able.

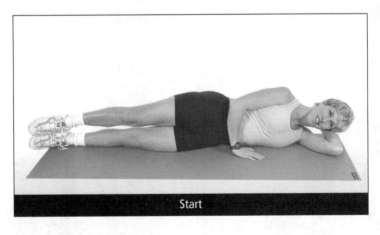

Start

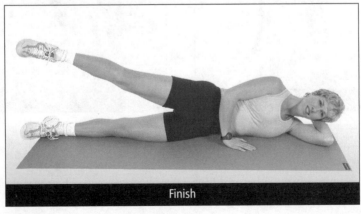

Finish

Advanced Outer-Thigh and Hip Toner**

- Assume an all-fours position with your knees and hands on the floor and your abdominal muscles tight. Keep your back straight.

- Keeping your leg bent, slowly raise your right leg to the side, away from the left leg.

- Slowly straighten and extend your right leg, hold, then bend the leg back slowly to the starting position.

- You will feel the work on the outside surface of your thigh, along the side of your leg and just below your butt.

- Complete 8 to 12 reps, then repeat on the other side.

- Add ankle weights as you're able.

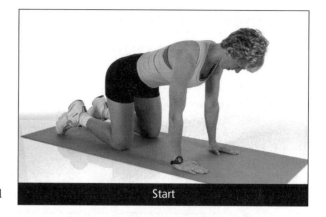

Start

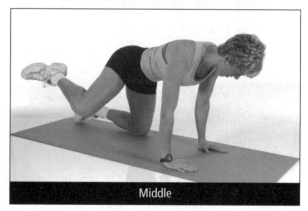

Middle

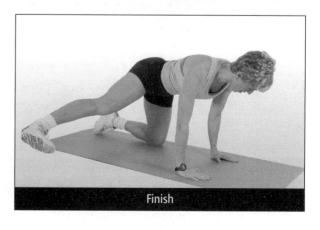

Finish

Inner-Thigh Toner

The inner-thigh toner helps firm and build muscle in the inner thigh.

Beginner Inner-Thigh Toner

- Lie on your right side with your leg, shoulder, and hips aligned.

- Bend your left leg and set it on the floor in front of you.

- Slowly lift your right leg, hold, and slowly lower it.

- You will feel the work on the inside of your thigh.

- Complete 8 to 12 reps, then repeat on the other side.

- Add ankle weights as you're able.

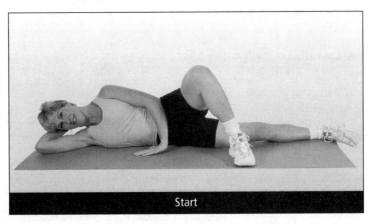

Start

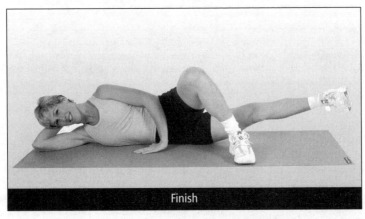

Finish

Advanced Inner-Thigh Toner (Frog Exercise)

- Lie on your back with your hands next to your buttocks, palms down.

- Tighten your abs, then bring your knees to your chest, keeping your feet together over your butt and letting your knees splay out.

- Slowly raise your legs straight up while pressing the inner surfaces of your feet together. Stop before your legs are completely straight, hold, and slowly lower your knees back to your chest.

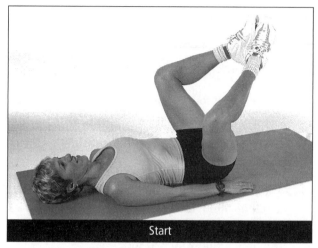

Start

- You will feel the work on the inside of your thigh.

- Complete 8 to 12 reps.

- Add ankle weights as you're able.

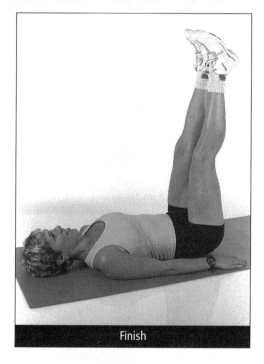

Finish

Back-of-Thigh and Buns Toner

The back-of-thigh and buns toner helps build muscle and improve tone in the back thighs and the butt.

Beginner Back-of-Thigh and Buns Toner**

- Assume an all-fours position with elbows and knees on the floor.

- Tighten your abs and straighten one leg.

- Raise your leg slowly straight toward the ceiling, hold, then slowly return to the floor. Be sure to keep your back straight, not allowing it to sag.

- You will feel this exercise work at the back of your lifted thigh and buns.

- Complete 8 to 12 reps, then repeat on the other side.

- Add ankle weights as you're able.

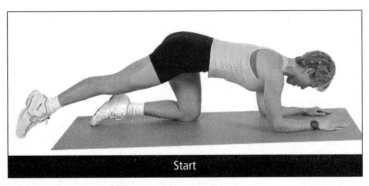

Start

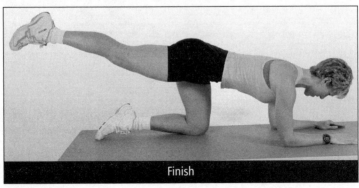

Finish

Advanced Back-of-Thigh and Buns Toner**

- Lie on your back and bend your left knee while keeping the foot flat on the floor. Your arms should rest on the floor.

- Set your right ankle on your left knee. Tighten your abs.

- Slowly lift your buns off the floor (about 4 to 6 inches) by squeezing your buns together tightly. Hold, and then slowly lower your buns toward the floor. Tap your buns down lightly, then repeat.

- Your left bun and back of left thigh should feel the work.

- Complete 8 to 12 reps, then repeat on the other side.

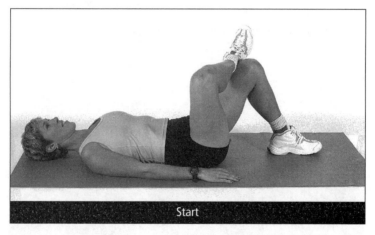
Start

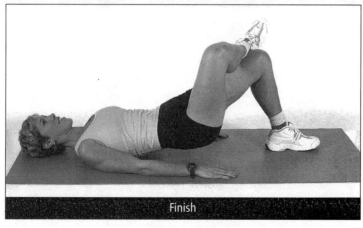
Finish

Upper-Abdominal Curls

Upper-abdominal curls help tone and build the upper abdomen.

Beginner Upper-Abdominal Curls**

- Lie on your back with your knees bent and your feet flat on the floor.

- Tighten your abs and flatten your back against the floor. Maintain a flattened back throughout the entire exercise.

- Interlace your fingers behind your neck.

- Slowly lift your shoulders off the floor, hold, and then slowly lower your shoulders to the floor. (Be careful not to "crank" on your neck.)

- Feel the work primarily along the upper portion of your abs, above the waist.

- Complete 8 to 12 reps.

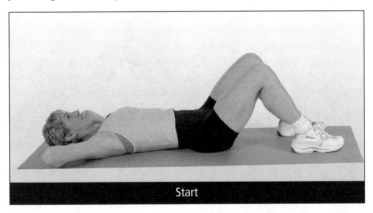

Start

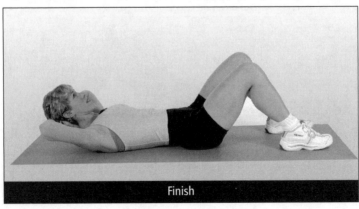

Finish

Advanced Upper-Abdominal Curls**

- Lie on your back with your knees bent and your feet flat on the floor.

- Tighten your abs and flatten your back against the floor. Maintain a flattened back throughout the entire exercise.

- Slowly raise your shoulders off the floor with arms extended, reaching to your knees with your hands, hold, then slowly lower your shoulders.

- You will feel the work primarily along the upper portion of your abs, above the waist.

- Complete 8 to 12 reps.

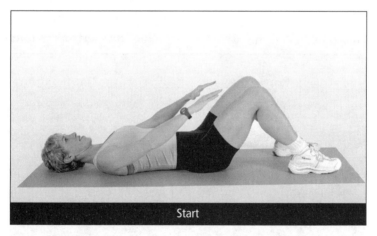

Start

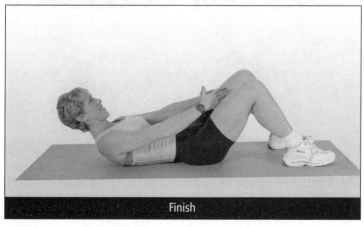

Finish

Diagonal Abdominals

Diagonal abdominals help tone and strengthen the sides of your waist.

Beginner Diagonal Abdominals**

- Lie on the floor and cross your left foot over your bent right knee.

- Tighten your abs and flatten your back against the floor.

- Interlace your fingers behind your neck.

- Slowly lift your right shoulder toward your left knee (but don't actually touch it), hold, then slowly lower your right shoulder.

- You will feel the work primarily along the left side of your abs (the oblique muscles).

- Complete 8 to 12 reps, then repeat on the other side (opposite abs will feel it).

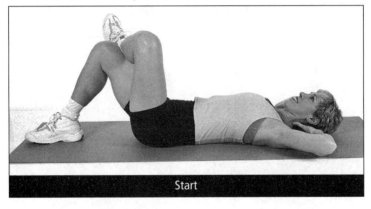

Start

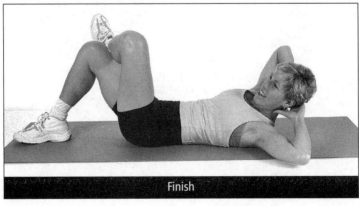

Finish

Advanced Diagonal Abdominals**

- Lie on the floor and bend your knees with your feet flat on the floor, then rest your knees so that they rotate and drop to the left side.

- Interlace your fingers behind your neck.

- Slowly lift your shoulders straight up off the floor, hold, and then slowly lower the shoulders.

- You will feel the work primarily along the left side of your abs (the oblique muscles).

- Complete 8 to 12 reps, then repeat on the other side (opposite abs will feel it).

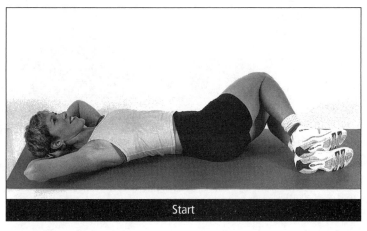

Start

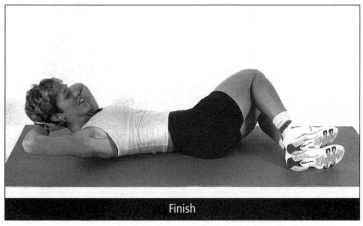

Finish

Step 4: Strength Training

Lower Abdominals

Lower abdominals tone and strengthen the abdominal area, primarily below the waist.

Beginner Lower Abdominals

- Lie on your back and place your hands under your buttocks, palms down.

- Bend your knees up at roughly a 90-degree angle, with your feet off the floor and ankles crossed.

- Tighten your abs muscles and flatten your back against the floor.

- Slowly lift your knees toward your chest, lifting your tailbone just a few inches off the floor, hold, then slowly lower your legs back to the starting position. Go slowly.

- You will feel this work on your abdominal muscles, primarily the lower abs, below the waist.

- Complete 8 to 12 reps.

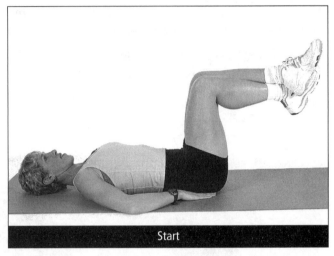

Start

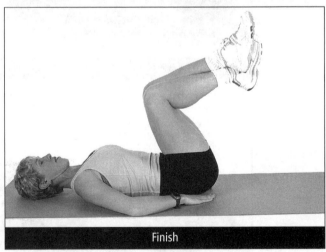

Finish

Advanced Lower Abdominals

- Lie on your back and place your hands under your buttocks, palms down.

- Lift your legs straight up in the air and cross them.

- Tighten your abdominal muscles and flatten your back against the floor.

- Now bring your legs toward your chest by tightening your lower abdominal muscles, hold, then return slowly to the starting position.

- You will feel the work primarily in the lower abs, below your waist.

- Complete 8 to 12 reps.

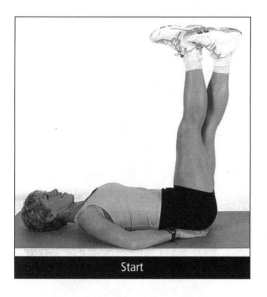
Start

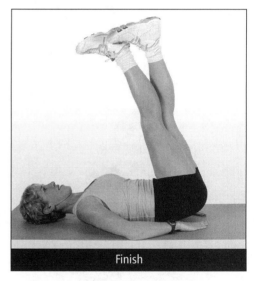
Finish

Upper-Arm Builder: Biceps Curls

Biceps curls help tone and strengthen the front of the upper arms.

- While sitting in a sturdy chair, grasp a medium-size hand weight in your left hand.

- Brace your left elbow against the inside of your left thigh.

- Slowly bend the elbow, curling the hand weight to just beyond 90 degrees, hold, and slowly lower the weight.

- You will feel the work on the inside of your upper arm.

- Complete 8 to 12 reps, then repeat on the other side.

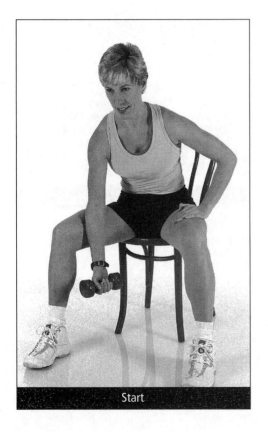

Start

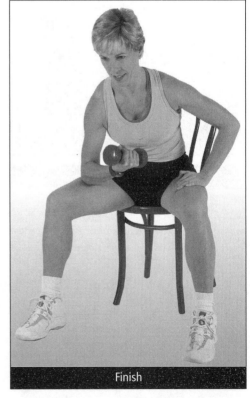

Finish

Upper-Arm Builder: Triceps Extension**

Triceps extensions help tone and strengthen the back of the upper arms.

Note: The advanced version of this exercise is the Level III upper-arm toner described on page 82.

- Lie on your back with your knees bent. Tighten your abdominal muscles.

- With a hand-held weight in each hand, bend your elbows so your hands are by your ears and your elbows are pointing toward the ceiling.

- Slowly straighten your arms, lifting the hand weight toward the ceiling. Stop before the arms are completely straight. Hold, then slowly lower the weights to the starting position.

- You will feel the work along the back of your upper arm.

- Complete 8 to 12 reps.

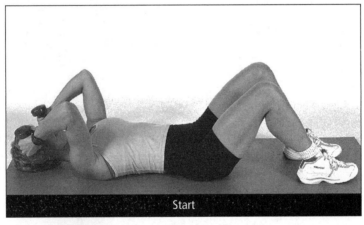
Start

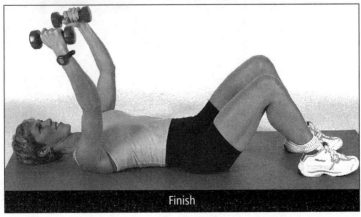
Finish

Upper-Back Builder: Bent-Over Arm Raise**

Bent-over arm raises tone and strengthen the upper-back muscles.

- Sit in a sturdy chair with a pillow on your lap. Grasp a small hand weight in each hand.

- Lean forward, keeping your back straight, with your arms at your sides.

- Keeping your elbows slightly bent, raise your arms to your sides, stopping just below shoulder level. Hold, then slowly lower the weights back down.

- You will feel the work along both sides of your upper back.

- Complete 8 to 12 reps.

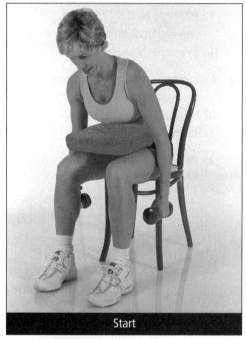

Start

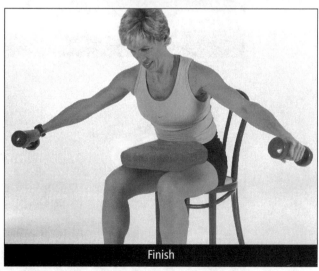

Finish

THE 15-MINUTE STRENGTH TRAINING PROGRAM

If you are pressed for time, we have a short workout for you to tone your body's major muscle groups. Be sure to perform at least 1 set of each exercise. These exercises provide a basic workout—the most effect in the least time. The 15-Minute Program is comprised of the following exercises (all of which were starred in the previous descriptions):

- thigh toners

- outer-thigh and hip toners

- back-of-thigh and buns toners

- upper-abdominal curls

- diagonal abdominals

- upper-arm builders: triceps extension

- upper-back builders

Do 1 set of each of these exercises at the appropriate level for you. Of course, the full program provides more benefit, but you will at least maintain your Strength Training program with this short workout.

Beginner Short Strength Training Program

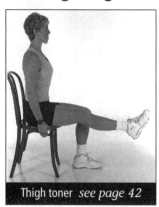

Thigh toner *see page 42*

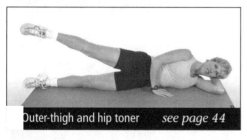

Outer-thigh and hip toner   *see page 44*

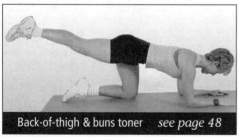

Back-of-thigh & buns toner   *see page 48*

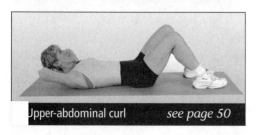

Upper-abdominal curl   *see page 50*

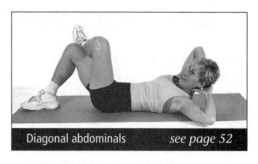

Diagonal abdominals   *see page 52*

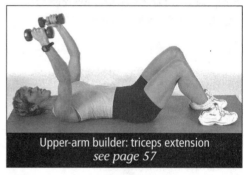

Upper-arm builder: triceps extension
see page 57

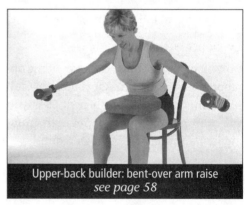

Upper-back builder: bent-over arm raise
see page 58

Advanced Short Strength Training Program

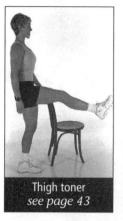

Thigh toner
see page 43

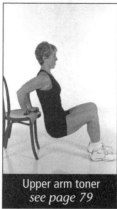

Upper arm toner
see page 79

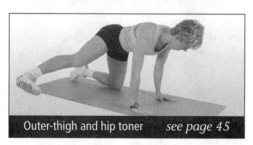

Outer-thigh and hip toner   *see page 45*

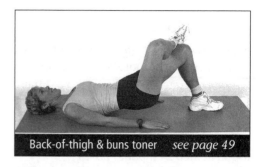

Back-of-thigh & buns toner   *see page 49*

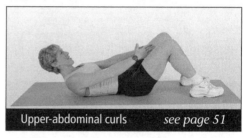

Upper-abdominal curls   *see page 51*

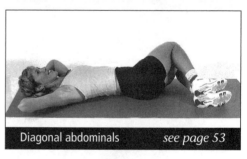

Diagonal abdominals   *see page 53*

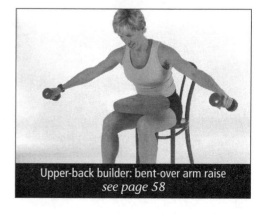

Upper-back builder: bent-over arm raise
see page 58

Step 4: Strength Training

Stretching

Regardless of which program you choose, remember to incorporate the four *Shape-Walking* stretches into your fitness program—ideally at the end of your workout when your muscles are still warm. Detailed descriptions of these stretches can be found in Step 2 on pages 20–21.

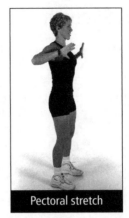

Pectoral stretch

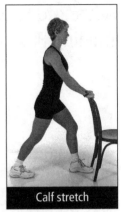

Calf stretch

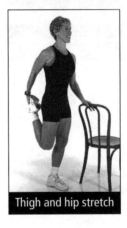

Thigh and hip stretch

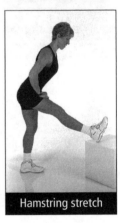

Hamstring stretch

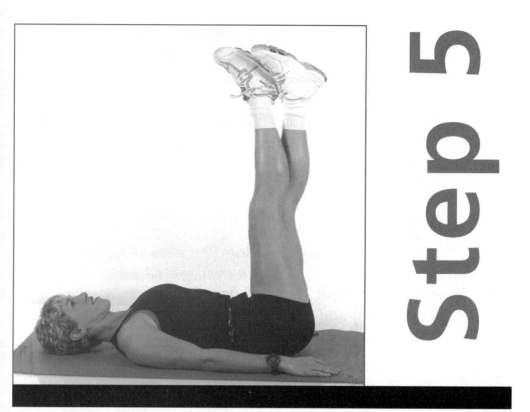

Target Toning

Target Toning (target muscle/muscle-group toning) is the third ingredient in *ShapeWalking's* Best-Body Formula. Target Toning provides extra emphasis on specific body-shaping trouble spots. It is also where the program gets the most personal.

Step 5: Target Toning

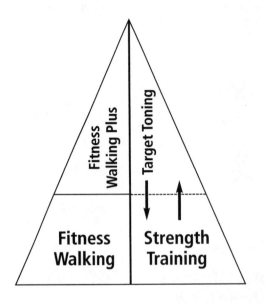

Fitness Walking Plus

Target Toning

Fitness Walking

Strength Training

Everybody needs the aerobic, calorie-burning benefits of Fitness Walking and the overall muscle-toning benefits of Strength Training, but your Target Toning needs are unique. Because no two bodies are alike, every person has special shaping needs.

Target Toning Needs

Amy

She just had her third child and her abdominal muscles know it. They are flabby and weak. Amy has also been feeling occasional lower-back pain, which is probably related to a lack of abdominal muscle tone.

Tom

He puts in long hours at a desk job and it is starting to show. An extra tire around the waist is now complemented by the beginnings of "desk-butt"—a wider and mushier rear end.

Marcy

She cannot locate a spot that doesn't need shaping. A slow weight gain of 2 to 3 pounds per year has added up to an extra 45 pounds. The added weight and an inactive lifestyle have left Marcy with a "doughy" appearance from too much fat and too little muscle tone.

Sheila

She's sick of her saddlebags, her biggest body-shaping blemish. She is hoping to find the right formula to trim her outer thighs and hips.

Target Toning Inventory

You know your own body and your body-shaping goals. Answer the following Target Toning Inventory to determine which Target Toning exercises will help you move toward your best body.

Abdomen

	YES	NO
Would you like your abdomen to be flatter?	___	___
Is your abdomen as tight and toned as you would like?	___	___
When you gain weight, does it "settle" in the middle?	___	___

> *If you answered yes to any of these questions, you could benefit from Target Toning exercises for the abdomen (see pages 67–71).*

Thighs

Is extra weight giving you a "pear" shape, with ample hips and thighs?	___	___
Do you hope to lose your saddlebags?	___	___
Do you have saggy knees—extra fat and skin that hang over your knees?	___	___
Has cellulite made its home in your thighs?	___	___

> *If you answered yes to any of these questions, you could benefit from Target Toning exercises for the thighs and hips (see pages 72–77).*

Buttocks

Do you feel "bottom heavy," with a butt that is wider and bigger than you want?	___	___
Are your buns flat instead of shapely?	___	___
Would you like your buttocks to be more firm and toned?	___	___

> *If you answered yes to any of these questions, you could benefit from Target Toning exercises for the buttocks (see pages 78–79).*

Upper Arms

Do your upper arms fatigue easily during house and yard tasks, such as carrying groceries and raking?	___	___
Are your upper arms flabby instead of firm?	___	___
Do you hate wearing sleeveless shirts because your upper arms are unattractive?	___	___

> *If you answered yes to any of these questions, you could benefit from Target Toning exercises for the upper arms (see page 80–82).*

Step 5: Target Toning

Target Toning Exercises

Target Toning exercises are designed to tone specific muscle/muscle groups to create a sleeker, sculpted look. The specific areas targeted are the following:

1. upper abs

2. lower abs

3. diagonal (side) abs

4. front thighs

5. outer thigh and hip

6. inner thighs

7. buttocks

8. upper arms

The names of these eight areas get mentioned frequently at the body-shape complaint department. Target Toning adds a little toning "oomph" to these bothersome trouble spots.

Principles

Target Toning is one element of your overall conditioning program. You still need the aerobic workout to burn calories and fat and the complete Strength Training program for balanced major-muscle-group conditioning. Target Toning, on the other hand, is frosting on the fitness cake—it sweetens the body-shaping program, but it must rest solidly on the other elements.

TARGET TONING GUIDELINES
For the entire Target Toning program use the following specific guidelines:
Frequency: 3 times per week
Reps: 12–15
Sets: Start with 1 set of each of Level I, Level II, and Level III exercises; work up gradually to 2–3 sets of each level.

Target Toning allows you to adapt the general Strength Training program to meet your personal, specific body shaping needs in a simple way. All of us need an overall balanced Strength Training program and a sound nutritional program. That's the point where toning must begin. Target Toning then adds a more focused toning approach to areas that need more work. If your saddlebags are making you sad, you can add Target Toning for the thighs and hips to the Strength Training program. If your gut has got you down, you can give it some added work with Target Toning for the abs.

While the general Strength Training program involves 1 or more sets of **1** exercise for each major muscle group, with Target Toning you will do 1 or more sets of **3** different exercises for each targeted muscle/muscle group. Doing three different exercises for one major muscle group gives these toning trouble spots a focused, varied, and more intense workout that tones and shapes the targeted area.

Target Toning involves many of the same exercises outlined in the Strength Training program plus some added advanced exercises. The Target Toning program presents exercises specifically for the eight trouble areas mentioned.

Form Matters

Carefully follow narrative and photos presented to help you perform the exercises correctly.

Be Consistent and Patient

Start easily and progress gradually. Be consistent. A regular schedule of Target Toning will yield much beter results than sporadic attempts. Be patient. It will take a few weeks to notice really significant differences in strength and tone.

Schedule

Target Toning should be done 3 times per week. You can do it 2 times per week with your regular Strength Training program and add 1 additional exercise session of only Target Toning on a different day. Or if you are already performing Strength Training 3 days a week, incorporate Target Toning into all 3 workouts. Just make sure there is a day off between Target Toning sessions.

Pick and choose the exercises that seem to get at your trouble spots most effectively. You can do as many of the Target Toning exercises as you wish, but be-cause they are fairly lengthy exercises, we recommend choosing no more than three or four at a time. To see results continue to work any Target Toning area for at least 6 weeks.

In order to help you plan your Target Toning program for the weeks ahead, make copies of the blank "Target Toning Progression Chart" on page 119.

Ab Toners

Most of us do not routinely tax our abdominal muscles during our normal daily activities. To trim your waist and tighten your abdominal muscles, you need a workout that challenges these muscles. The *ShapeWalking* Target Toning program for your abs does just that.

Where to Start

- If you have pouching at the top of the abdomen, work the upper abdominals.

- If your 18 year old waist is lost along with your high school jeans, emphasize the diagonal/side abdominals, which work the oblique muscles.

- If your lower abdomen has softened due to prenancy and birth or just life, select the lower abdominals. (See illustration on page 26.)

The first three exercises are for the abdominal major muscle groups (for more

Step 5: Target Toning

on these muscles see pages 25–27). Choose one or all of them.

Principles

For maximum results, keep the following points in mind as you Target Tone your abdominals:

Form Matters

It is hard to think of any exercises where form matters more than it does for abdominal muscles. Three simple tips can assure effectiveness and safety:

1. Flatten your back against the floor and maintain that position throughout the entire set of repetitions. This will protect your lower back from stress and strain and maximally challenge the abdominal muscles.

2. Go slowly. Move in a controlled manner. Ballistic and erratic movements can cause injury and limit the challenge to the abdominal muscles. Start with a count of 2 in the lifting phase, hold for 2 counts, and return to the starting position to a 2 count. Progress to a 4 count up, 4 hold, and 4 down. Quality matters far more than quantity.

3. It is very tempting to hold your breath when your abdominal muscles are working, but you should breathe normally throughout the exercises.

Be Consistent and Patient

Start easily and progress gradually. Be consistent. A regular schedule of abdominal toning will yield much better results than sporadic attempts. Be patient. It will take a few weeks to notice really significant differences in strength and tone.

How Much, How Often

Start with one set of 12–15 reps of each of the three exercises—Levels I, II, and III. Work up to 2–3 sets of 12–15 reps for each of the three exercises.

Exercises that are already described in the general Strength Training program are starred. You can turn to the list of pages for a detailed description of these exercises.

SUMMARY OF TARGET TONING GUIDELINES

1. Target Tone only two areas during any 6-week period.
2. Use correct form.
3. Start at the right level.
4. Perform the complete program.
5. Be consistent and patient.

Frequency: 3 times per week

Reps: 12 to 15

Sets: 3

Count: initially 2 counts per phase with a long-range goal of 4 counts per phase (lifting, holding, returning to start)

Upper Abdominals: Levels I and II

Start with the Level I and II exercises that are actually repeats of the exercises on pages 50 and 51 (photos showing the "Finish" position for these two exercises are reproduced here for easy reference). After completing these exercises, move on to the Level III exercise below.

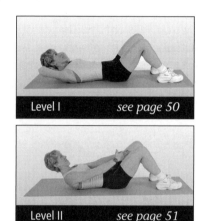

Upper Abdominals: Level III

- Lie on your back with your knees bent and your feet flat on the floor.

- Tighten your abs and flatten your back against the floor. Maintain a flattened back throughout the entire exercise.

- Grasp a handheld weight in both hands and reach overhead, extending your arms just beyond your head. Do not allow your back to arch up.

- Slowly raise your shoulders off the floor, hold, and then slowly lower your shoulders.

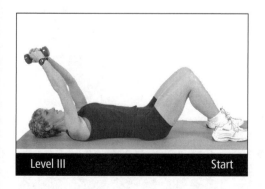

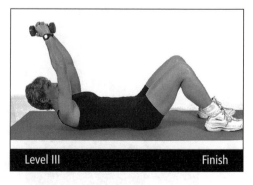

Step 5: Target Toning

Lower Abdominals: Levels I and II

Start with the Level I and II exercises that are actually repeats of the exercises on pages 54 and 55 (photos showing the "Finish" position are reproduced here for easy reference). After completing these exercises, move on to the Level III exercise shown at the bottom of this page.

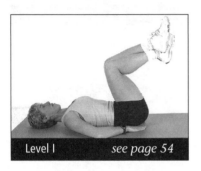

Level I   *see page 54*

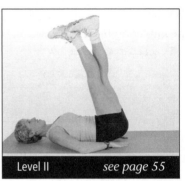

Level II   *see page 55*

Lower Abdominals: Level III

- Lie on your back and place your hands under your buttocks, palms down.

- Tighten your abdominal muscles and flatten your back against the floor.

- Lift your legs straight up in the air.

- Now slowly lower your legs toward the floor. Stop between 30 and 45 degrees from straight up. Hold, and slowly bring your legs back to the straight up position. Your back should not arch up at all.

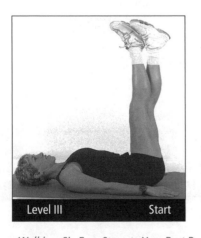

Level III   Start

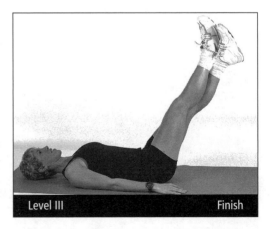

Level III   Finish

Diagonal/Side Abdominals: Levels I and II

Start with the Level I and II exercises that are actually repeats of the exercises on pages 52 and 53 (photos showing the "Finish" positions are reproduced here for easy reference). After completing these exercises, move on to the Level III exercise below.

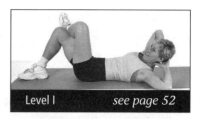

Level I   *see page 52*

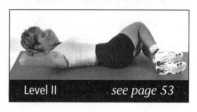

Level II   *see page 53*

Diagonal/Side Abdominals: Level III

- Lie on your back with your knees bent up 90 degrees at the hips and 90 degrees at the knees. Your arms should lie palms down next to your sides.

- Tighten your abdominal muscles and flatten your back against the floor.

- Slowly rotate your knees 45 degrees

to one side, hold, then return to the middle. Now repeat on the other side.

- Continue alternating side to side until you have completed 1 set.

- Be sure to maintain the angle at the hips. You will be tempted to "cheat" by bringing your knees closer in toward your chest.

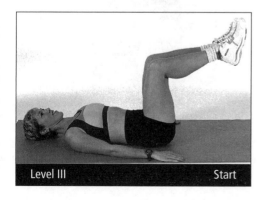

Level III   Start

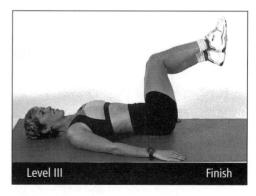

Level III   Finish

Thigh Toners

The following exercises are designed to turn your soft, squishy upper legs into solid, sleek muscles that will support all your life's activities

Where to Start

- If the front of your thighs are squishy, do the Front-Thigh exercises.

- If you look in the mirror and see unwanted curves high on the sides of your legs, jump into the Outer-Thigh and Hip routines.

- If your inner thighs meet as you walk down the street, begin with the Inner-Thigh toners.

For triple duty you can eventually tackle all three areas during your workout for super toning.

Front-Thigh Toner: Level I

Start with the Advanced Thigh Toner exercise on page 43 (photo showing the "Finish" position is reproduced here for easy reference). After completing this exercise, move on to the Level II and III exercises on the next two pages.

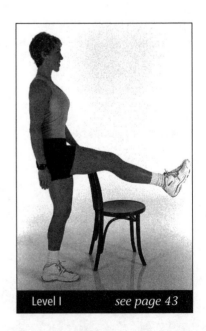

Level I   *see page 43*

Front-Thigh Toner (Squat): Level II

- Stand in front of a chair with feet hip-width apart and feet parallel.

- Bend your knees and sit back so that your buns are nearly touching the seat of the chair.

- Bring your arms up and point them forward 90 degrees (arms parallel to the floor).

- Hold, then use the front thigh muscles to return slowly to the starting position.

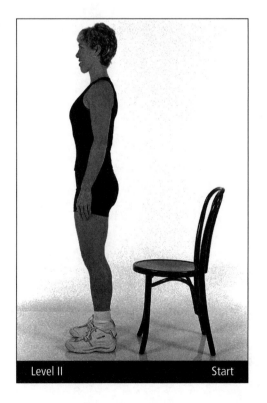

Level II   Start

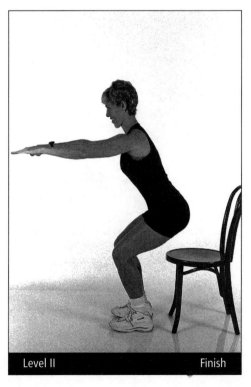

Level II   Finish

Front-Thigh Toner (Lunge): Level III

- Stand upright with your feet about 6 inches apart, toes pointed straight ahead.

- Step forward with your right foot as far as possible, bending your left knee as you do. Continue this motion until

your left knee almost touches the floor, hold, then slowly return to the starting position.

- Do 1 set; then repeat on the opposite side.

- Add hand weights as you're able.

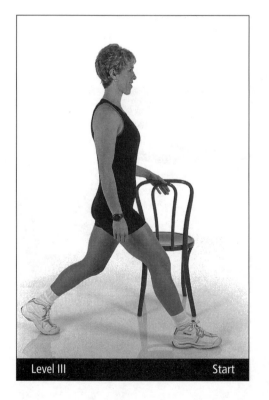

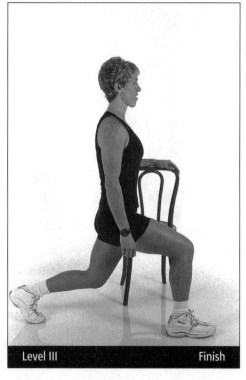

Outer Thigh and Hip Toner: Levels I and II

Start with the Level I and II exercises that are actually repeats of the exercises on pages 44 and 45 (photos showing the "Finish" positions are reproduced here for easy reference). After completing these exercises, move on to the Level III exercise below.

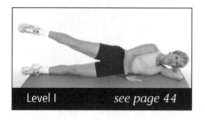

Level I   *see page 44*

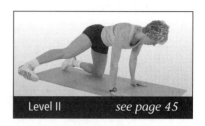

Level II   *see page 45*

Outer-Thigh and Hip Toner: Level III

- Lie on your back. Tie a length of resistance band around your knees quite snugly.

- Bend your knees, keeping your feet flat on the floor. Place your arms at your sides and your feet shoulder-width apart.

- Tighten your abdominal muscles. Now squeeze your buttocks and lift them off the floor so that your knee, hip, and shoulder are aligned.

- While maintaining this alignment, slowly open your knees outward against the resistance band, hold, and slowly bring the knees back. Do not allow the hips to sink.

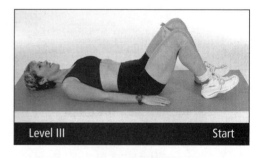

Level III   Start

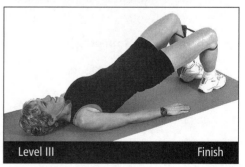

Level III   Finish

Inner-Thigh Toner: Level I

Start with the Level I exercise that is actually a repeat of the exercise on page 46
(photo showing the "Finish" position is reproduced here for easy reference). After
completing this exercises, move on to the
Level II exercise below.

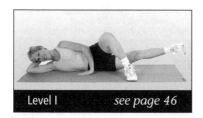

Level I — *see page 46*

Inner-Thigh Toner: Level II

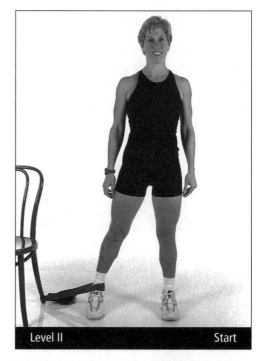

Level II — Start

- Tie a resistance band around your
  right ankle. Fasten the other end of the
  band to a stationary object (chair,
  etc.). Stand with feet hip-width apart.

- Pull your right foot toward your left
  foot, keeping feet parallel.

- You will feel the work on the inside of
  your right thigh.

- Complete 12 to 15 reps.

- Repeat with the other foot.

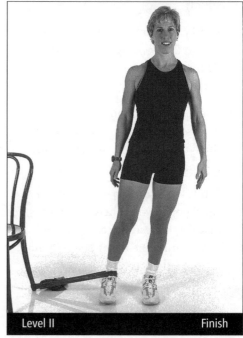

Level II — Finish

Inner-Thigh Toner (Frog Exercise): Level III

The Level III exercise is a repeat of the exercise described in detail on page 47 (photos of both the "Start" and "Finish" positions are reproduced here for easy reference).

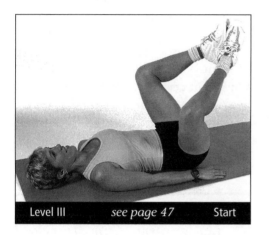

Level III *see page 47* Start

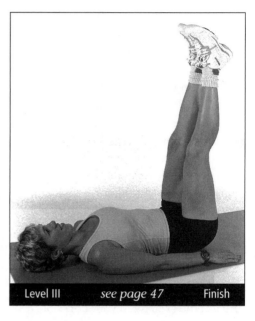

Level III *see page 47* Finish

Step 5: Target Toning

Buttocks Shape Up

If you are looking for a better rear view—a tight and shapely tush—try the Target Toning buttocks exercises. Enhance the effectiveness of this program by contracting your gluteal muscles (squeezing your cheeks together) frequently during the day—during work meetings, while sitting at traffic lights, during commercials.

For maximum results, keep these points in mind as you do the buttocks toners.

Focus Your Efforts

Concentrate on using the buttocks to power you through the movements. Know what it feels like to work this muscle and focus on doing so. Keep your cheeks tight throughout the entire exercise. Go slowly and feel the exercise in your backside.

Hold Your Form

Keep your back straight throughout each exercise. Do not let it sag or arch.

How Much, How Often

Do your buttock Target Toning exercises 3 times per week. Remember, a repetition is a complete movement, from start to finish and back to starting again, and a set is the number of reps you perform continuously. Start with 1 to 2 sets of 5 to 10 repetitions with the beginner Target Toning exercises. Work up to 3 sets of 12 to 15 reps. Then add 1 set of 12 to 15 reps with the intermediate toning exercises. (You are now doing 1 set of intermediate and 2 sets of beginner.) When that gets easy, add 1 set of 12 to 15 reps with the advanced toning exercises. You are now doing 1 set at each level. This variety of exercises will give maximum toning results.

SUMMARY OF BUTTOCKS TARGET TONING GUIDELINES

Frequency: 3 times per week

Reps: 12 to 15

Sets: 3

Count: initially 2 counts per phase with a long-range goal of 4 counts per phase (lifting, holding, returning to start)

Buttocks Tightener: Levels I and II

Start with the Level I and II exercises that are actually repeats of the exercises on pages 48 and 49 (photos showing the "Finish" positions are reproduced here for easy reference). After completing these exercises, move on to the Level III exercise below.

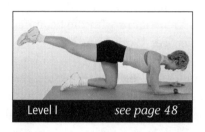

Level I   *see page 48*

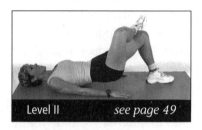

Level II   *see page 49*

Buttocks Tightener (Single-Leg Bridge): Level III

- Lie on your back and bend your knees with your feet flat on the floor. Your arms should rest on the floor.

- Straighten your left leg so that both knees are parallel.

- Slowly lift your buns off the floor so that your knee, hip, and shoulder are aligned. Hold and slowly lower.

- You will feel the work mainly in the right buttocks.

- Complete 12 to 15 reps, then repeat on the other side.

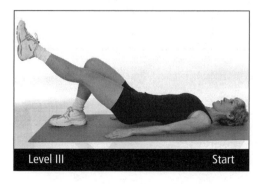

Level III   Start

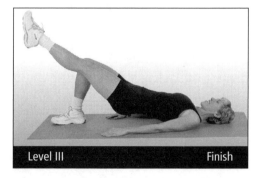

Level III   Finish

Step 5: Target Toning

Upper-Arm Firmers

The triceps along the back of the upper arm are one of the most underused muscles in the body. By contrast, the biceps along the front of the upper arm are used whenever you carry or lift objects. Because they are frequently weak, the triceps are often flabby and jiggle when you move. The Target Toning upper-arm program is the answer to your wiggling, jiggling upper arms.

For maximum results, keep the following points in mind as you tone your upper arms.

Keep It Under Control

Swinging weights around wildly won't do anything to eliminate flabby upper arms. Keep the exercises under control. Go slowly.

Finish with a Stretch

After your upper-arm workout is complete, follow it up with the Pectoral stretch (see page 20). This will relieve any tension present in your shoulder muscles.

How Much, How Often

Do your upper-arm Target Toning exercises 3 times per week. Remember that a repetition is a complete movement, from start to finish and back to starting again, and a set is the number of reps you perform continuously. Start with 1 to 2 sets of 5 to 10 repetitions with the beginner toning exercises. Work up to 3 sets of 12 to 15 reps. Then add 1 set of 12 to 15 reps with the intermediate toning exercises. (You are now doing 1 set of intermediate and 2 sets of beginner). When that gets easy, add 1 set of 12 to 15 reps with the advanced toning exercises. You are now doing 1 set at each level. This variety of exercises will give you maximum toning results.

SUMMARY OF UPPER-ARM TARGET TONING GUIDELINES

Frequency: 3 times per week

Reps: 12 to 15

Sets: 3

Count: initially 2 counts per phase with a long-range goal of 4 counts per phase (lifing, holding, returning to start)

Upper-Arm Toner: Level I

Start with the Level I exercise that is actually a repeat of the exercise on page 57 (photo showing the "Start" and "Finish" positions are reproduced here for easy reference). After completing this exercises, move on to the Level II exercise below.

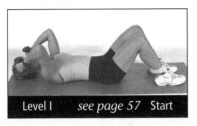

Level I   *see page 57*   Start

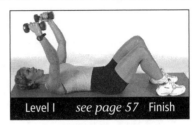

Level I   *see page 57*   Finish

Upper-Arm Toner: Level II

- Stand with one foot in front of the other. Lean forward, placing your left hand on the seat of a firm chair.

- While holding a medium weight in your right hand, bring your elbow back.

- Keeping your elbow stationary, slowly straighten your lower arm, hold, then slowly bend the elbow back again.

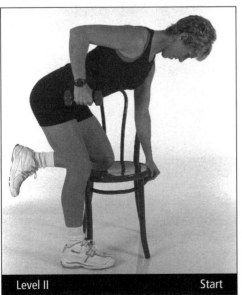

Level II   Start

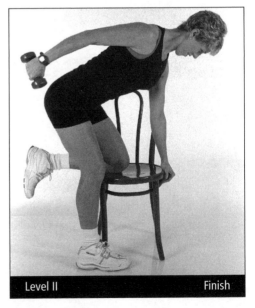

Level II   Finish

Upper-Arm Toner: Level III

- Place your hands on the seat of a chair behind you. Keep your legs bent at a 90-degree angle.

- Keeping your back straight, slowly bend your elbows to about 90 degrees, hold, then slowly straighten your elbows again.

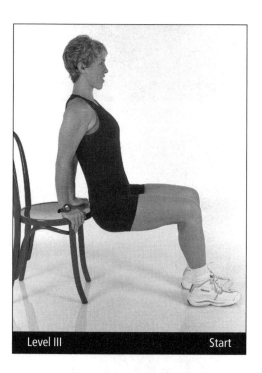

Level III   Start

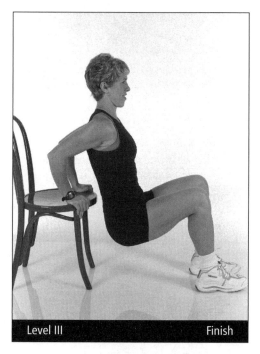

Level III   Finish

Use this Target Toning program to hit your body-shaping trouble spots. In a few short weeks, these areas should be slimmer and tighter. Remember to stretch at the end of each workout. Your best body is closer than you think!

Stretching

Remember to incorporate the four *Shape-Walking* stretches into your fitness program—ideally at the end of your work-out when your muscles are still warm. Detailed descriptions of these stretches can be found in Step 2 on pages 20–21.

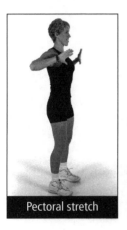
Pectoral stretch

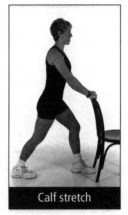
Calf stretch

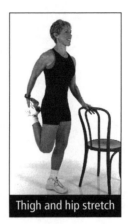
Thigh and hip stretch

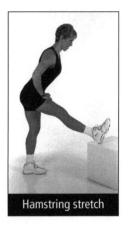
Hamstring stretch

Your Notes:

· ·

· ·

· ·

· ·

· ·

· ·

· ·

· ·

· ·

· ·

· ·

· ·

· ·

· ·

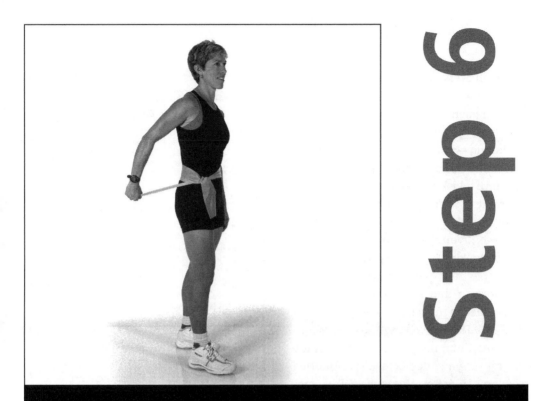

A Week in the Life of a *ShapeWalker*

What does a week of *ShapeWalking* look like? Because no two people have the exact same body-shaping needs, *ShapeWalking* will look different for each person.

Step 6: A Week in the Life of a *ShapeWalker*

Although every person's *ShapeWalking* program is and should be different, the principal ingredients—Fitness Walking, Fitness Walking Plus, Strength Training, and Target Toning—will always be the foundation of an effective body-shaping program.

Since a lack of time is the number-one deterrent to sticking with an exercise program, we also offer the option of active housework/yardwork as an alternative to Fitness Walking if you are pressed for time. Guidelines for performing housework/yardwork so that it "counts" as exercise are detailed in the section "Everyday Alternatives to Fitness Walking" on page 88.

A brief summary of each aspect of the program is presented below. It is followed by examples of how the *ShapeWalking* program is used by four different people with varying body-shaping goals.

FITNESS WALKING AND FITNESS WALKING PLUS

Frequency: most, if not all, days of the week

Start with: as long a walk as you can, while maintaining a fast pace and good form

Long-term goal: three 45–60 minute walks and two 30-minute walks each week

Helpful hints: use proper form to move faster and burn more calories

Add Fitness Walking Plus: for added toning to the abs, buttocks, thighs, or upper arms

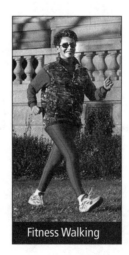

Fitness Walking

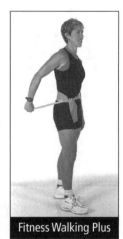

Fitness Walking Plus

STRENGTH TRAINING

Frequency: 2 to 3 times each week

Start with: the beginner-level exercise, at a minimum of 1 set of 8, 10, or 12 repetitions, counting 2 for each move (2 up, 2 hold, 2 down)

Goal: advancing in level and weights as you're able to, 2 sets per exercise

Helpful hint: Substitute Target Toning exercises for your trouble spots. (For example, do the Target Toning ab program instead of the Strength Training abdominal program if this is your trouble spot. The Target Toning program is more intense.) If you are pressed for time, do the 15-minute short Strength Training program. Whenever you can, perform the full 30-minute Strength Training program. If you want more of a challenge, increase to 4 counts for each phase.

TARGET TONING

Frequency: 3 times each week

Start with: 1 set each of Levels I, II, and III, with 12 to 15 repetitions

Goal: 2–3 sets each of Levels I, II, and III

Helpful hint: Adapt the program as you need to so that you are adequately challenged.

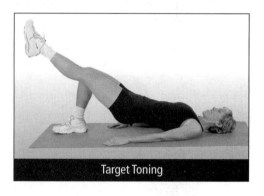

Target Toning

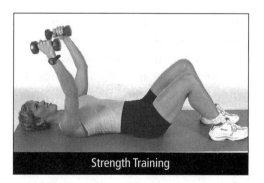

Strength Training

Stretching

The *ShapeWalking* stretching program is just four simple stretches (see exercises on pages 20–21). Each stretch is designed to address a flexibility "hot spot"—an area particularly prone to loss of range of motion. Do this stretching after you finish your workout for the day, regardless of which parts of the program you do: Fitness Walking, Fitness Walking Plus, Strength Training, or Target Toning. The time you inves in stretching will be 2 minutes and 40 seconds well spent.

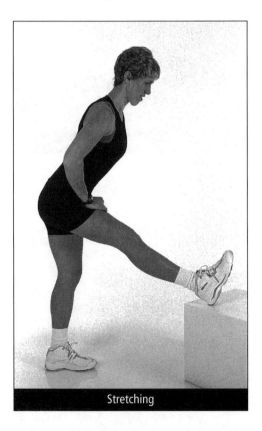
Stretching

Everyday Alternatives to Fitness Walking

A lack of time is the number-one deterrent to sticking with an exercise program. When the kids need you and work is calling and the lawn needs mowing and the dishes are stacked up, it is really hard to convince yourself that 30 minutes of Fitness Walking is the right priority. Fortunately, *ShapeWalking* does allow you to substitute 30 to 45 minutes of fairly vigorous yard or housework for a Fitness Walking session once or twice a week.

You might not be used to thinking of raking leaves and picking up around the house as exercise, but these activities require rhythmic, repetitive movement and muscular effort. They have the potential to work your aerobic system and tone your muscles. Anyone who has woken sore and stiff after a day of spring housecleaning or fall yardwork knows that these activities can challenge your fitness level. When you substitute house and yardwork for Fitness Walking, you can keep your body-shaping goals on track *and* simultaneously tackle some necessary household chores.

Some simple qualifications must be met before household tasks count as exercise. First, you need to *keep moving at a pretty good pace.* Some casual sweeping and slow, easy raking will not do. You need to move as if you really mean to get it done. Clean like company's coming in a few minutes. Mow and rake like you need to get it done before a storm rolls in shortly.

The second qualification is to keep this pace up for the entire "exercise" session. If you were scheduled for a 20-minute Fitness Walk, do 20 minutes of chores. If you were scheduled for a 45-minute walk, do 45 minutes of chores. Sometimes, especially with housework, this might require some planning. It doesn't take 45 minutes to sweep the kitchen floor. For shorter duration tasks, you must string together enough of them to fill up your time allotment.

For example, Mary was set to walk 35 minutes, but was so stressed out about the state of her house that she decided to substitute 35 minutes of vigorous housework. She planned to start with picking up, then vacuuming, and finally sweeping. She got the vacuum and broom out—and off she went. Moving quickly from room to room and up and down the stairs, Mary got everything picked up. Without a pause she moved on to vacuuming, pushing it back and forth at a good clip. Finally, she grabbed the broom and finished with some vigorous sweeping. When she was done, Mary was slightly winded and her heart was beating faster. She got a 35-minute workout—and a cleaner house.

The final qualification for exercise is that the tasks chosen must be at least moderately physically vigorous. Washing and drying dishes do not qualify—they are too easy to be considered exercise. Here is a list of tasks around the house and

yard that do qualify as exercise and can be substituted for Fitness Walking.

Moderately vigorous

- sweeping
- vacuuming and picking up
- carrying in and quickly unloading groceries
- gardening

Very vigorous

- washing windows
- landscaping
- raking
- mowing with a push lawn mower
- shoveling snow by hand

In summary, to qualify as exercise, house and yard chores must

- be done at a quick pace
- be done for the entire duration without rest
- be at least moderately physical

To help you design your *ShapeWalking* schedule, pages 90–93 show four examples of schedules that suit individuals with different goals.

Step 6: A Week in the Life of a *ShapeWalker*

Liz's Week of *ShapeWalking*

Liz came to *ShapeWalking* because it meets two important fitness-program criteria for her: It is inexpensive and it can be done at home. Having gone the health-club route in the past, Liz knew she was much more likely to stick with a program if she did not have to get in her car and drive somewhere.

Now, confronting middle age, Liz made a renewed commitment to improved health and fitness. She found she could no longer get away with the "eating and exercise sins of youth." Now when she ate too much fatty food or played couch potato too long, it showed—right on her hips. Liz set the following three goals when she started *ShapeWalking*:

1. to feel better and have more energy

2. to lose 20 pounds

3. to get rid of her saddlebags

Liz went on her first Fitness Walk 6 months ago. She barely made 15 minutes that day, but she stuck with the program faithfully and can now do over 3 miles in 45 minutes. She has made great strides toward achieving all three of her fitness goals. After 6 months on the program, this is what a week of *ShapeWalking* looks like for Liz.

Liz gets four walks in, choosing to add Fitness Walking Plus for her thighs during three of the walks. She substitutes 45 minutes of moderately vigorous housework for one long walk and gets a workout while getting a cleaner house. Liz does Target Toning for the outer thighs and hips, which she completes 3 times. Finally, she also does her overall strengthening program twice.

	FITNESS WALKING	FITNESS WALKING PLUS	STRENGTH TRAINING	TARGET TONING	STRETCHING
MON	30 minutes	thighs		outer thighs and hips	2 min. 40 sec.
TUE	45 minutes	thighs			2 min. 40 sec.
WED	45 minutes		30 minutes	outer thighs and hips	2 min. 40 sec.
THU	substitute 45 minutes of housework				
FRI	day off—evening with friends				
SAT	30 minutes	thighs	30 minutes		2 min. 40 sec.
SUN	35 minutes			outer thighs and hips	2 min. 40 sec.

Tom's Week of *ShapeWalking*

Tom is new to *ShapeWalking*. He started the program 4 short weeks ago. He is still gradually increasing his walking times, working toward the goal of 30 to 45 minutes each day. As a computer programmer, Tom spends 8 or more hours each day at a desk. He has gradually gained 30 pounds, all of which seems to have landed around his waist. Tom is also the father of two preschoolers, so time is precious at home. Tom chose *ShapeWalking* because he can accomplish the major part of the program at work by walking during his lunch hour. He does the Strength Training and Target Toning exercises while watching the news after tucking the little ones into bed each night. Below is what a week of *ShapeWalking* looks like for Tom.

Tom includes five Fitness Walking outings, each 20 to 25 minutes in length, as he works gradually toward his goal of Fitness Walking 30 to 45 minutes daily. He does Fitness Walking Plus at work during all of his walks, so he efficiently gets the benefit of toning as well as an aerobic workout. He Target Tones his abs intensely by performing Target Toning for the upper, diagonal, and lower abs 3 times, as well as performing the full Strength Training program twice during the week.

	FITNESS WALKING	FITNESS WALKING PLUS	STRENGTH TRAINING	TARGET TONING	STRETCHING
MON	20 minutes	abs	30 minutes	upper, diagonal, and lower abs	2 min. 40 sec.
TUE	22 minutes	abs			2 min. 40 sec.
WED	22 minutes	abs	30 minutes	upper, diagonal, and lower abs	2 min. 40 sec.
THU	23 minutes	abs			2 min. 40 sec.
FRI	25 minutes	abs		upper, diagonal, and lower abs	2 min. 40 sec.
SAT	day with family				
SUN	day with family				

Step 6: A Week in the Life of a *ShapeWalker*

Jodi's Week of *ShapeWalking*

Jodi has one fitness goal—looking great. For Jodi, this means being thin and toned. She chose *ShapeWalking* because she was looking for a program that focused on the areas that matter the most for a great shape—the abs, thighs, and upper arms. Jodi enjoys Fitness Walking, but she is definitely more focused on the Strength Training and Target Toning exercises. Most people choose only two areas to Target Tone per session. However, Jodi does not see herself as "most people." We have all seen Jodi diehards at the gym. Below is what a week of *ShapeWalking* looks like for Jodi.

Jodi does 5 days of Fitness Walking, alternately adding the toning benefits of Fitness Walking Plus. Three days per week she does the Strength Training program as well as Target Toning for the upper and diagonal abs; the front thighs and inner thighs; the buttocks; and arms. She especially enjoys the intense Target Toning sessions, when she tones the areas she feels need the most work and that make her look her best when they are toned.

	FITNESS WALKING	FITNESS WALKING PLUS	STRENGTH TRAINING	TARGET TONING	STRETCHING
MON	30 minutes	arms/abs 4 spots	full minus		2 min. 40 sec.
TUE	30 minutes	thighs/buttocks		abs/thighs/ buttocks/arms	2 min. 40 sec.
WED			full minus 4 spots		2 min. 40 sec.
THU	30 minutes	arms/abs		abs/thighs/ buttocks/arms	2 min. 40 sec.
FRI	30 minutes	thighs/buttocks	full minus 4 spots		2 min. 40 sec.
SAT	30 minutes	arms/abs		abs/thighs/ buttocks/arms	2 min. 40 sec.
SUN	day off				

Andrea's (Always Stressed for Time) Week of *ShapeWalking*

Occasionally all of us experience unusually busy weeks. Rather than slacking off exercise at these times, do the best you can to exercise at a minimal maintenance level. You will feel better and maintain your progress, even when you are at your busiest. Below is what a week of *Shape-Walking* looks like for Andrea.

During Andrea's busy week she fits in three 30-minute Fitness Walking outings as well as two 30-minute alternatives to Fitness Walking—housework and yardwork. She also finds time for two sessions of the 15-minute short Strength Training program. These minimal activities help her maintain her level of conditioning.

	FITNESS WALKING	FITNESS WALKING PLUS	STRENGTH TRAINING	TARGET TONING	STRETCHING
MON	30 minutes				2 min. 40 sec.
TUE	30 minutes housework/ yardwork		15-minute short program		2 min. 40 sec.
WED	30 minutes				2 min. 40 sec.
THU	30 minutes housework/ yardwork		15-minute short program		2 min. 40 sec.
FRI	day off				
SAT	30 minutes				2 min. 40 sec.
SUN	day off				

Step 6: A Week in the Life of a *ShapeWalker*

Your Week of *ShapeWalking*

To help you develop your own *ShapeWalking* program, here is a blank calendar for your use. You may want to make multiple photocopies of the blank form in case your schedule or needs change as you progress with your program.

	FITNESS WALKING	FITNESS WALKING PLUS	STRENGTH TRAINING	TARGET TONING	STRETCHING
MON					
TUE					
WED					
THU					
FRI					
SAT					
SUN					

Some Words About Weight Loss

It has long been reported that the winning formula for losing weight is sensible, healthful eating and increased physical activity. Because it is easy and inexpensive, *ShapeWalking* is an ideal way to increase activity and burn more calories and fat. Here are some simple modifications to the *ShapeWalking* program to make it an even more potent way to lose weight.

Increase the Length of Your Fitness Walking Outings

Set a goal of walking 45 to 60 minutes most, if not all, days of the week. These longer outings result in more calories burned and more weight lost.

Increase the Intensity of Your Fitness Walking

Work to increase overall speed while walking. Or add some speed intervals by increasing walking speed from fast to very, very brisk for a set amount of time or distance. For example, if you are on a 45-minute walk, incorporate speed intervals by picking up the pace and walking as fast as you can for 1 minute at each 5-minute interval. Alternatively, add hills or stairs to increase the intensity.

Add the Fitness Walking Plus Elements

Fitness Walking Plus is designed to address some specific body-toning trouble spots, but everyone can add these elements to their Fitness Walk. As a result, your muscles will get some extra toning, which, in turn, burns more calories and fat.

Do Strength Training 3 Times Per Week

By doing 3 days of Strength Training (instead of the minimum of 2 outlined in the *ShapeWalking* program), you get more muscle toning. Remember, the more muscle tone you have, the more fat and calories you burn.

ShapeWalking also offers these five important tips for healthy, sensible eating.

1. Drink More Water

Many people commonly confuse hunger with thirst, so they eat unneeded food when they really need something to drink. Water is the healthful drink of choice. It has no calories, no fat, and no chemicals. Drinking water also lends a sense of fullness, which diminishes cravings for food. Also, as you increase your activity level, water becomes even more important. Drink a minimum of eight 8-ounce glasses of water per day (you may count juice, herbal teas, other noncaffeinated fluids, or soup toward your eight glasses).

2. Eat More Vegetables

Vegetables are a very filling low-calorie food. They are high in fiber, which makes you feel full by providing bulk. In addition, vegetables are an important source of vitamins and minerals.

3. Don't Skip Meals

Skipping meals is a form of deprivation, and the body reacts by strongly craving food, so skipping meals has a negative effect. Eating breakfast is especially important. Many experts consider skipping breakfast a major deterrent to successful weight loss. Instead of skipping meals, eat smaller, healthful portions at each meal. Supplement meals with small portions of healthful snacks.

4. Keep a Food Journal

Studies have repeatedly reported that writing down what you eat is an effective tool for changing eating habits and losing weight. Purchase a small notebook and write down everything you eat every day.

5. Shop Smarter

Since most of us eat the majority of our meals at home or from lunches prepared at home, changing eating habits begins with shopping smarter. If rich, fatty foods are not in your house, you are less likely to eat them.

Begin by making a menu for each meal. Buy all the ingredients you will need to make easy, healthful meals. Develop a list and stick with it. Be sure to put several low-fat, healthful snacks on your shopping list. Focus your purchases on healthful choices such as fresh produce, low-fat dairy, lean meat, whole grains, and legumes.

Dealing with Boredom

The secret to alleviating boredom when you exercise is to add variety. Fortunately, that is very easy to do with Fitness Walking. Since you are not tied to a certain room or a specific piece of equipment, you have the freedom to vary several elements.

Begin by choosing a new place to walk. Treat yourself by driving to a trail near a lake or park once a week. You might also try walking at a different time of day. If you are a morning walker, walk in the evening, or if the evening is your usual time, try the afternoon.

Signing up for a walking race can be a huge motivator. With a race scheduled, it is time to kick into training mode. It is easier to get out the door and walk a little longer and a little harder when you know your abilities will be tested in a race.

You might also consider joining a walking club or finding a buddy to walk with you on some days. Not only will this help hold you to a scheduled time and place to walk, but conversation can also make the workout time go by faster. Also, try vigorous new aerobic activites such as the elliptical trainer, a treadmill set at a challenging incline, or a fun class such as kickboxing.

Overcoming Plateaus

The longer you work the *ShapeWalking* program (or any other fitness program), the more likely you are to hit a plateau. Hitting a plateau simply means that progress toward your fitness goals has temporarily leveled off. It means you're doing the same work without seeing the same results.

Although plateaus are a normal event on the fitness journey, you can do some things to shorten them. One of the greatest contributors to fitness and weightloss plateaus is doing the same workout over and over. Try adding some variety. Change Fitness Walking courses to make the work more challenging. Repeatedly walk up and down any hills on the course or add some quicker-paced time intervals by walking at an accelerated pace for 1 to 2 minutes at a time.

Also, try varying your Strength Training routine. Change the order of the exercises you are doing or try different exercises for any given body area.

Sometimes rest is the right prescription for busting plateaus. If your workout has gotten monotonous, take 3 or 4 days off. You will likely jump back in with new energy and enthusiasm after a short rest.

Most of all, be patient. As long as you are working hard and challenging yourself, you will get through a plateau with time. Set your sights on your body-shaping goals and keep plugging away.

ShapeWalking for Life

A lifetime of fitness is a very worthwhile goal. No matter how old you are or how fit you may be, you can start right now to get fit for life. Wherever the road may take you over the years, take *ShapeWalking* with you.

ShapeWalking has all the elements you need for a complete fitness program at any age. Fitness Walking can challenge your fit body if you move fast and maintain good form. Over the years, as you age, you can simply adapt Fitness Walking to your changing abilities. Your pace may slow and your stride may shorten, but walking will still be an easy and effective route to fitness, even with advancing age.

The Strength Training and Target Toning programs can also be adapted to age-related changes in ability. Initially, Strength Training and Target Toning are

Step 6: A Week in the Life of a *ShapeWalker*

often seen as important routes to a better body shape. Later, with advancing age, Strength Training also becomes a critical means of maintaining physical function. Improved strength allows the older adult to maintain a life of activity and independence.

Start now to make *ShapeWalking* a part of your daily life. This highly adaptable program can meet your body-toning and fitness goals now—and for a lifetime.

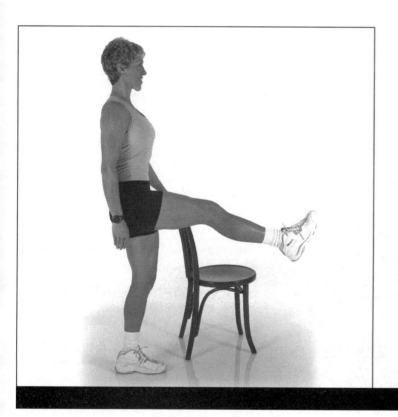

Overview of the Exercises

Now you have seen how four individuals with different fitness goals are using the *ShapeWalking* program. To help you design your own program, the following section presents a brief overview of all of the exercises in this book.

Fitness Walking

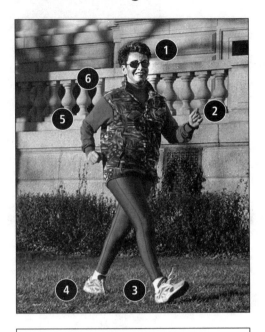

FITNESS WALKING AND FITNESS WALKING PLUS

Frequency: most, if not all, days of the week

Start with: as long a walk as you can, while maintaining a fast pace and good form

Long-term goal: three 45–60 minute walks and two 30-minute walks each week

Helpful hints: use proper form to move faster and burn more calories

Add Fitness Walking Plus: for added toning to the abs, buttocks, thighs, or upper arms

REMEMBER TO

1. Stand tall with head up
2. Keep hands in a loose fist
3. Land on your heel
4. Push with your toe
5. Bend elbows 90 degrees, keeping them close to the body and swinging
6. Keep shoulders slightly back and relaxed

Fitness Walking Plus

Add special toning exercises for your abs, thighs, buttocks, or upper arms to Fitness Walking most if not all days of the week.

For Abs

Hold your abdominal muscles tight, sucking them into your belly button while you walk.

1. tighten your muscles until they fatigue

2. take a 2-minute rest

3. retighten your muscles

4. take a 2-minute rest

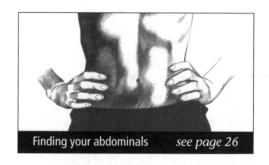

Finding your abdominals   *see page 26*

For Buttocks

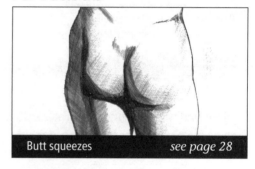

Butt squeezes   *see page 28*

For Thighs

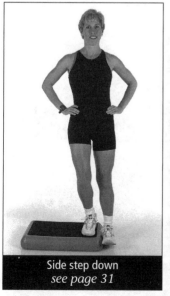

Side step down
see page 31

For Thighs

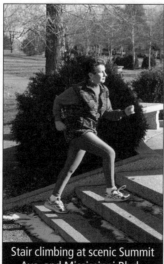

Stair climbing at scenic Summit Ave. and Mississippi Blvd., St. Paul, Minnesota *see page 32*

For Arms

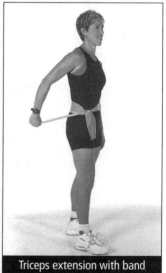

Triceps extension with band
see page 33

Strength Training

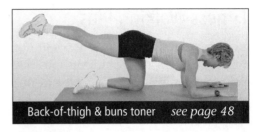

Back-of-thigh & buns toner   *see page 48*

STRENGTH TRAINING BEGINNER SHORT PROGRAM
Frequency: 2 to 3 times each week, but not 2 days in a row
Start with: the beginner-level exercise shown
With the goal of: advancing in level and weight, as much as you are able
Reps: 8 to 12 per set
Sets: at least 1 set per exercise, preferably 2 sets per exercise
Count: start with 2 counts for each phase; progress to 4 counts for each phase

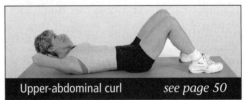

Upper-abdominal curl   *see page 50*

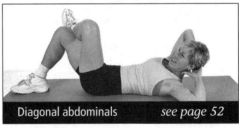

Diagonal abdominals   *see page 52*

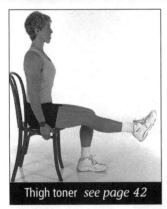

Thigh toner *see page 42*

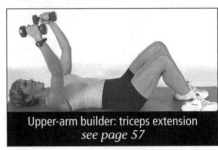

Upper-arm builder: triceps extension
see page 57

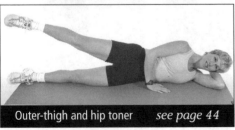

Outer-thigh and hip toner   *see page 44*

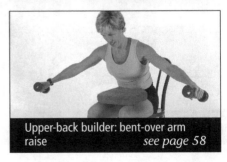

Upper-back builder: bent-over arm raise   *see page 58*

STRENGTH TRAINING BEGINNER FULL PROGRAM

When time permits, add the following exercises to the seven exercises that make up the short program.

Frequency: 2 to 3 times each week, but not 2 days in a row

Start with: the beginner-level exercise shown

With the goal of: advancing in level and weight, as much as you are able

Reps: 8 to 12 per set

Sets: at least 1 set per exercise, preferably 2 sets per exercise

Count: start with 2 counts for each phase; progress to 4 counts for each phase

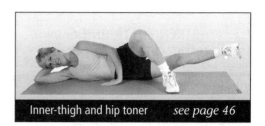
Inner-thigh and hip toner   *see page 46*

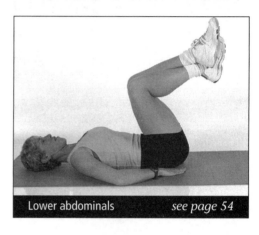
Lower abdominals   *see page 54*

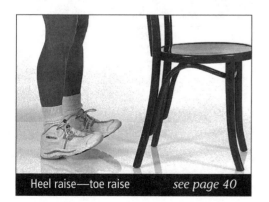
Heel raise—toe raise   *see page 40*

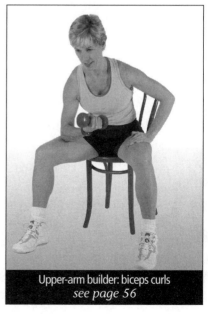
Upper-arm builder: biceps curls
see page 56

Overview of the Exercises

STRENGTH TRAINING ADVANCED SHORT PROGRAM

Progress to the advanced level gradually. You should have been doing the beginner program for at least 6 weeks before moving on to the advanced program.

Frequency: 2 to 3 times each week, but not 2 days in a row

With the goal of: advancing in level, as much as you are able

Reps: 8 to 12 per set

Sets: at least 1 set per exercise, preferably 2 sets per exercise

Count: start with 2 counts for each phase; progress to 4 counts for each phase

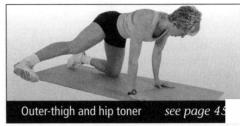
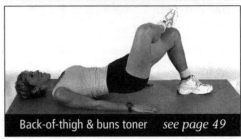

Outer-thigh and hip toner *see page 45*

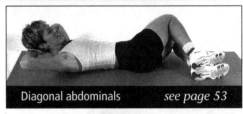

Back-of-thigh & buns toner *see page 49*

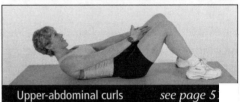

Upper-abdominal curls *see page 5*

Diagonal abdominals *see page 53*

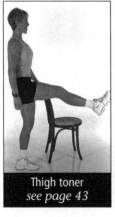

Thigh toner
see page 43

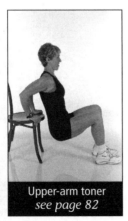

Upper-arm toner
see page 82

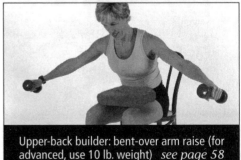

Upper-back builder: bent-over arm raise (for advanced, use 10 lb. weight) *see page 58*

STRENGTH TRAINING ADVANCED FULL PROGRAM

When time permits, add the following exercises to the seven exercises that make up the short program.

Frequency: 2 to 3 times each week, but not 2 days in a row

With the goal of: advancing in level, as much as you are able

Reps: 8 to 12 per set

Sets: at least 1 set per exercise, preferably 2 sets per exercise

Count: start with 2 counts for each phase; progress to 4 counts for each phase

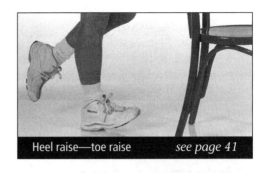

Heel raise—toe raise   *see page 41*

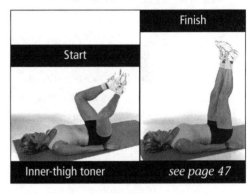

Start   Finish

Inner-thigh toner   *see page 47*

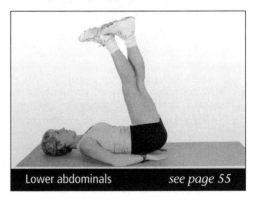

Lower abdominals   *see page 55*

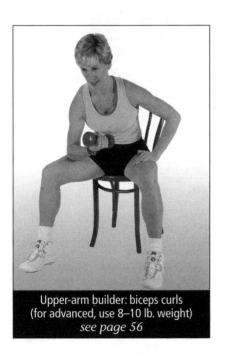

Upper-arm builder: biceps curls
(for advanced, use 8–10 lb. weight)
see page 56

GENERAL TARGET TONING GUIDELINES

1. To guide you to which trouble spots to work on, take the Target Toning Inventory on page 65.
2. Work on just 3 or 4 areas at a time.
3. Work consistently on these areas for at least 6 weeks before changing areas.
4. **Frequency:** 3 times per week
5. **Reps:** 12–15
6. **Sets:** Start with one set each of Level I, Level II, and Level III exercises; work up gradually to 2–3 sets of each level.
7. Continue aerobic conditioning by taking 3 45-minute and 2 30-minute Fitness Walks per week.
8. Follow a sound nutritional plan aimed at achieving an appropriate body weight for you. Seek nutritional guidance if needed.

Target Toning: Abdominals

Upper Abdominals

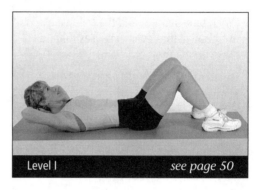

Level I   *see page 50*

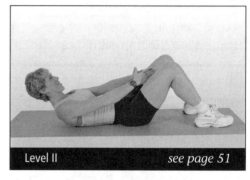

Level II   *see page 51*

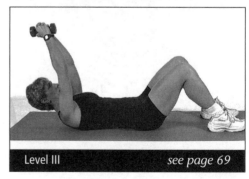

Level III   *see page 69*

Lower Abdominals

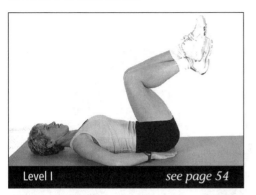

Level I   *see page 54*

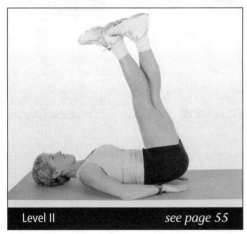

Level II   *see page 55*

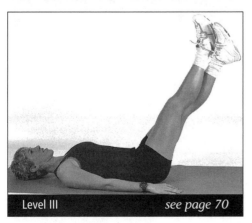

Level III   *see page 70*

Diagonal Abdominals

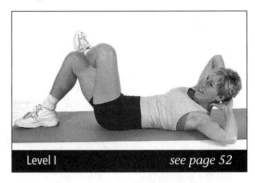

Level I   *see page 52*

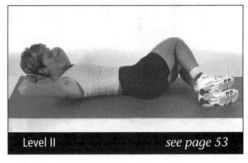

Level II   *see page 53*

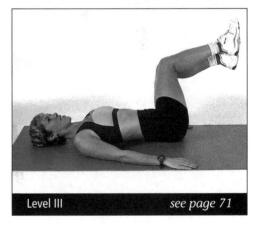

Level III   *see page 71*

Target Toning: Thighs

Front Thigh

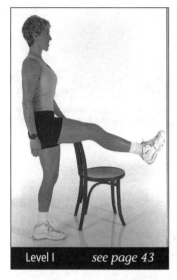

Level I   *see page 43*

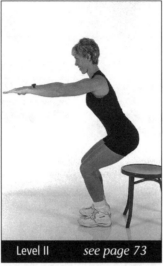

Level II   *see page 73*

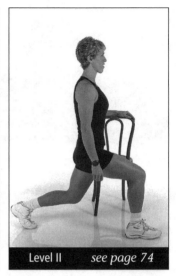

Level II   *see page 74*

Outer Thigh and Hip

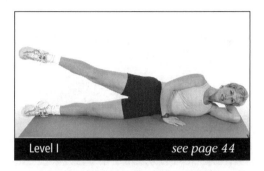

Level I   *see page 44*

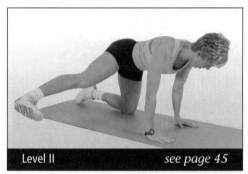

Level II   *see page 45*

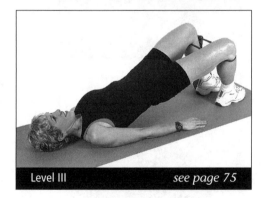

Level III   *see page 75*

Inner Thigh

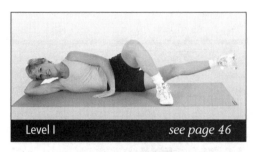

Level I   *see page 46*

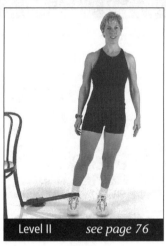

Level II   *see page 76*

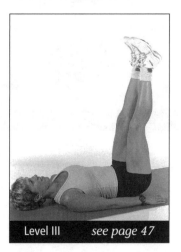

Level III   *see page 47*

Overview of the Exercises

Target Toning: Buttocks

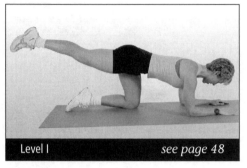

Level I   *see page 48*

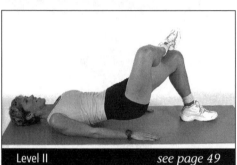

Level II   *see page 49*

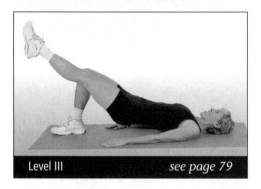

Level III   *see page 79*

Target Toning: Upper Arms

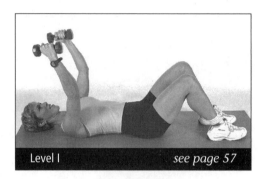

Level I   *see page 57*

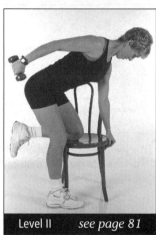

Level II   *see page 81*

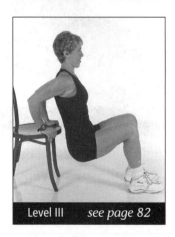

Level III   *see page 82*

Conclusion

Congratulations! By reaching this point you have made major positive strides toward achieving your best body. If you've been practicing the *ShapeWalking* program a step at a time, you might already feel a difference in the fitness of your body along with an improved mood and positive outlook. If you have just read straight through the book and have not yet begun to practice *ShapeWalking*, you still have gained an overview of the program.

No matter how old you are or how fit you may be, you can start right now to get fit for life and work toward your best body. The healthful, convenient, and low-cost *ShapeWalking* program has all the elements you need for a complete fitness program you can use for the rest of your life.

You have taken **Step One—Making the Decision to Shape Up**—by reading this book and perhaps beginning the exercises themselves. Every day you participate in *ShapeWalking* you are making the decision to develop and keep your best body.

Step Two—Fitness Walking—is as close as your shoes and the front door and as long lasting as your future. Fitness Walking can challenge your fit body if you move fast and maintain good form. Over the years, as you age, you can simply adapt Fitness Walking to your changing abilities. Your pace may slow and your stride may shorten, but walking will still be an easy and effective route to fitness, even with advancing age.

Step Three—Fitness Walking Plus—may appeal to you most just now. The Plus gives you that extra emphasis you need to work for an all-over toned and fit body. Once you see the results of Fitness Walking Plus you will want to keep your body in its best shape for a lifetime.

Steps Four and Five—Strength Training with Stretching and Target Toning—are initially seen as important routes to a better body shape. Later, Strength Training and Stretching can be adapted to age-related changes in ability and also may become critical means

Conclusion

of maintaining physical function. Improved strength and range of motion allow the older adult to maintain a life of activity and independence, and Target Toning continues to shape the areas that we notice most.

Step Six—The Weekly Plan—will carry you through the busy times and the slow times, from young adulthood through retirement. No matter your lifestyle, a lifetime of fitness can be managed easily in daily increments.

Add *ShapeWalking* to your daily life starting today. This highly adaptable program can help you to meet your body-shaping and fitness goals now—and for a lifetime. And a lifetime of fitness is a very worthwhile goal. Wherever the road may take you over the years, take *ShapeWalking* with you.

Appendix A: Heart Rate

Developing your best body requires exercising with enough intensity to make a difference. Chapter 2 describes three methods to determine if you are in the target zone of intensity—the talk test, the perceived exertion scale, and a simple heart-rate scale. All three methods work fine, but if you want to find your exact heart rate, simply follow these instructions.

To determine the specific heart-rate numbers for your target zone, first find your maximum heart rate. The maximum heart rate (MHR) equals 220 minus your age in years.

MHR = 220 – age (in years)

A target zone needs a low end and a high end. The low end is defined as 65 percent of the MHR and the high end is defined as 85 percent of the MHR. To find the lower limit, multiply your maximum heart rate by 0.65.

Lower limit (heartbeats per minute) = MHR x 0.65

To find the upper limit of the target zone, multiply your MHR by 0.85

Upper limit (heartbeats per minute) = MHR x 0.85

Exercising in "the zone" will keep your body-shaping and weight-loss goals on target. You can figure your exact zone using these instructions with your age or you can use a table. For simplicity's sake, we have determined the lower and upper limits for certain ages. Choose the age you are closest to and use the target zone outlined below.

TARGET ZONE BY AGE	
AGE	TARGET ZONE (HEARTBEATS PER MINUTE)
20	130 to 170
30	123 to 161
40	117 to 153
50	110 to 144
60	104 to 136
70	97 to 127

Taking Your Pulse

To determine how fast your heart is beating, you need to take your pulse. While you are exercising, slow down and quickly find your pulse. Use the tips of your index and middle fingers to find your pulse at the wrist or neck. Don't use the thumb; it has a pulse of its own. Look at your watch and take your pulse for 10 seconds, counting the number of heartbeats that occur in that amount of time. Multiply this number by six to determine the number of heartbeats per minute.

Appendix A: Heart Rate

Remember Sharon with the target zone of 117 to 153 heartbeats per minute? She took her 10-second pulse during a walk—it was 20.

Beats in 10 seconds x 6 = heartbeats per minute

It might be helpful for you to predetermine what the range is for your 10-second pulse. This is simply what your 10-second heart rate should be to stay in the target zone. Because it eliminates multiplying by 6, the 10-second pulse may be the easiest way to monitor walking intensity. To arrive at this number, divide the lower and upper limits of your target-zone heart rate by 6.

Most people find it easiest to use the 10-second target zone chart for certain ages. Just use the numbers for the age you are closest to.

TEN-SECOND TARGET ZONE	
AGE	TEN-SECOND PULSE RATE (HEARTBEATS PER 10 SECONDS)
20	22 to 28
30	21 to 27
40	20 to 26
50	18 to 24
60	17 to 23
70	16 to 21

Appendix B: Blank Worksheets

The blank worksheets on the next four pages will help you plan your own personalized fitness program. You may want to make photocopies in case you change your plan along the way.

- Fitness Walking Record

- Fitness Walking Plus Progression Chart

- Strength Training Progression Chart

- Target Toning Progression Chart

ShapeWalking Fitness Walking Record

Record the time or miles you spend in your target zone each day. Work up gradually—increase your time or miles at a rate of approximately 10 percent per week. Be sure to include two rest days per week in your program (A rest day could be walking at a pace below your target zone or engaging in any form of low- to moderate-intensity activity.)

	SUNDAY	MONDAY	TUESDAY	WEDNESDAY	THURSDAY	FRIDAY	SATURDAY
GOAL							
Week #1							
Week #2							
Week #3							
Week #4							
Week #5							
Week #6							
Week #7							
Week #8							
Week #9							
Week #10							

ShapeWalking Fitness Walking Plus Progression Chart

Choose from toning exercises for the abdominals, buttocks, upper arms, and thighs. You can do all the exercises on a single outing, or do different ones each day of the week. Work up gradually.

EXERCISE	SUNDAY		MONDAY		TUESDAY		WEDNESDAY		THURSDAY		FRIDAY		SATURDAY	
	Reps	Sets	Reps	Sets	Reps	Sets	Reps	Sets	Reps	Sets	Reps	Sets	Reps	Sets
Abs														
Butt Squeeze														
Triceps Extension with Band														
THIGHS														
Side Step Down														
Hills														
Stairs														

ShapeWalking Strength Training Progression Chart

If you are a novice, start with the beginner program. Begin with the weight that you have determined for your starting level. Do the exercises you have chosen for 8 repetitions (reps). When you can do 8 reps easily, increase to 10 reps, and finally to 12 reps. Once you can do 12 reps easily, move to the next weight and start at 8 reps again. Follow this progression for each exercise. After a minimum of 6 weeks, repeat the process for advanced-level exercises. On days when you are pressed for time, do the short program; otherwise do the full program. Perform your Strength Training program a minimum of two times per week—preferably three times. Photocopy this chart for you personal record keeping. **Always warm up before performing exercises. Always perform exercises with good form. NOTE: If at any time you feel pain while performing a particular exercise, STOP doing that exercise.**

EXERCISE	SUNDAY			MONDAY			TUESDAY			WEDNESDAY			THURSDAY			FRIDAY			SATURDAY		
	WGT.	REPS	SET	WGT.	REPS	SET	WGT.	REPS	SET	WGT.	REPS	SET	WGT.	REPS	SET	WGT.	REPS	SET	WGT.	REPS	SET
Thigh toner																					
Outer-thigh & hip toner																					
Back-of-thigh & buns toner																					
Upper-abdominal curls																					
Diagonal abdominals																					
Upper-arm builder																					
Upper-back builder																					
Biceps curls																					
Heel raise—toe raise																					
Lower abdominals																					
Inner-thigh toner																					

◄—— SHORT PROGRAM ——►
◄—— FULL PROGRAM ——————————————————►

ShapeWalking Target Toning Progression Chart

Use the Inventory on page 65 to choose 3 or 4 areas to emphasize. Begin with 1 set of your chosen areas at each level (I, II, and III), and gradually increase to 2–3 sets of each level for each Target Toning area.

DAY	ABDOMINALS			THIGHS			BUTTOCKS	UPPER ARMS
	Upper	Lower	Diagonal	Front	Outer-Hip	Inner		
SUNDAY								
MONDAY								
TUESDAY								
WEDNESDAY								
THURSDAY								
FRIDAY								
SATURDAY								

Bibliography

A Report of the Surgeon General. *Physical Activity and Health*. Pittsburgh, PA: Department of Health and Human Services, 1996.

American College of Sports Medicine (ACSM). *ACSM Guidelines for Exercise Testing and Prescription,* 5th Edition. Philadelphia, PA: Williams and Wilkins, 1995.

American College of Sports Medicine (ACSM). *ACSM Resource Manual for Guidelines for Exercise Testing and Prescription,* 3rd Edition. Baltimore, MD: Williams and Wilkins, 1998.

American College of Sports Medicine (ACSM). *Exercise Management for Persons with Chronic Diseases and Disabilities.* Champaign, IL: Human Kinetics, 1997.

American College of Sports Medicine (ACSM), position stand. "The Recommended Quantity and Quality of Exercise for Developing and Maintaining Cardiorespiratory and Muscular Fitness in Healthy Adults." *Medicine and Science in Sports and Exercise*, 22,2:265–274, April 1990.

American College of Sports Medicine (ACSM), position stand. "The Recommended Quantity and Quality of Exercise for Developing and Maintaining Cardiorespiratory and Muscular Fitness and Flexibility in Healthy Adults." *Medicine and Science in Sports and Exercise*, 30:975–91, 1998.

American Council on Exercise (ACE). *Personal Trainer Manual.* San Diego, CA: ACE, 1996.

Anderson, Robert A., and Jean E. Anderson. *Stretching*. Bolinas, CA: Shelter Publications, Inc., 1980.

Austin, Denise. *Hit the Spot: How to Target, Tone, and Slim Your Problem Areas*. New York: Simon & Schuster, 1997.

Baechle, Tom, and Barney Groves. *Weight Training—Steps to Success.* Champaign, IL: Human Kinetics Publishers, 1992.

Braverman, Susan P., Editor, *Review of Dietetics: Manual for the Registered Dietician Exam, 2000-2002 Edition.* Angel Fire, NM: Hess and Hunt, Inc., 2000.

Bricklin, Mark, and Susan G. Berg. *The Best of Prevention*. Emmaus, PA: Rodale, Inc., 1997.

Brooks, Douglas. *Effective Strength Training.* Mammoth Lakes, CA: Moves International Fitness, 2001.

Busch, Felicia. *The New Nutrition: From Antioxidants to Zucchini.* New York: John Wiley & Sons, Inc., 2000.

"Calories Go, Fast or Slow." *Walker's World.* 1997:5.

Clark, Nancy. "Fluids, Dehydration and Thirst Quenchers." Brookline, MA: Sports Medicine Brookline.

Clark, Nancy. *Sports Nutrition Guidebook.* Champaign, IL: Human Kinetics, 1997.

Convertino, V.A., et al., *Exercise and Fluid Replacement,* American College of Sports Medicine (ACSM) position stand, 1996.

Cook, Brian B., and Gordon W. Stewart. *Strength Basics.* Champaign, IL: Human Kinetics, 1996.

Cowles, Sage. *Fitness Walking Workshop.* Reebok Bodywalk. St. Paul, MN: SweatShop, 1996.

Cruise, Jorge. *8 Minutes in the Morning.* Emmaus, PA: Rodale, Inc., 2001.

The Editors of *Prevention Magazine. Women's Health Today 2002.* Emmaus, PA: Rodale, Inc., 2002.

Gerber, Niklaus J., and Bernhard Rey. "Can Exercise Prevent Osteoporosis or Reverse Bone Loss? A Review of Controlled Longitudinal Trials." *Physiotherapy: Controlled Trials and Facts.* 14:47–60, 1991.

Grant, Roberta. "Walk Off Weight this Winter." *Fitness.* Jan.–Feb., 1997: 40–44.

Green, Bob, and Oprah Winfrey. *Make the Connection: Ten Steps to a Better Body—and a Better Life.* New York: Hyperion, 1996.

Gutin., B., and M.J. Kasper. "Can Vigorous Exercise Play a Role in Osteoporosis Prevention? A Review." *Osteoporosis International.* 2:55–69, 1992.

Hurley, Ben. "Strength Training in the Elderly to Enhance Health Status." *Medicine, Exercise, Nutrition, and Health.* 4:217–229, 1995.

Iknolan, Therese. *Fitness Walking.* Champaign, IL: Human Kinetics Publishers, 1995.

Itjelm, Rick, P.T. "Brrr... Exercising Outdoors in Winter." *Sideline View.* Minneapolis, MN: The Institute of Athletic Medicine at Fairview Hospital, 1988.

Kannus, P., H. Sievanen, and I. Vuori. "Physical Loading, Exercise, and Bone." *Bone.* 18, 1:S1–S3, 1996.

Larson, Kate. *The LifeWalk Audio Training Program.* www.katelarsen.com. 2000.

Meyers, Casey. *Walking: A Complete Guide to the Complete Exercise.* New York: Random House, 1992.

Nelson, Miriam E., with Sarah Wernick. *Strong Women Stay Young.* New York: Bantam Books, 1997.

Bibliography

Otis, Carol, with Linda Lynch. "How to Keep Your Bones Healthy." *The Physician and Sportsmedicine.* 22, 1:71–72, 1994.

Oyster, Nancy, Max Morton, and Sheri Linnell. "Physical Activity and Osteoporosis in Postmenopausal Women." *Medicine and Science in Sports and Exercise.* 16,1:44–50, 1984.

The Editors of Prevention Health Books for Women. *Banish Your Belly, Butt & Thighs Forever!* Emmaus, PA: Rodale, Inc., 2000.

Sharkey, Brian J. *Fitness and Health.* Champaign, IL: Human Kinetics, 1997.

Simkin, Ariel, Judith Ayalon, and Isaac Leichter. "Increased Trabecular Bone Density Due to Bone-Loading Exercises in Postmenopausal Osteoporotic Women." *Calcified Tissue International.* 40:59–63, 1987.

Sinaki, Mehrsheed, and Kenneth P. Offord. "Physical Activity in Postmenopausal Women: Effect on Back Muscle Strength and Bone Mineral Density of the Spine." *Archives of Physical Medicine and Rehabilitation.* 69:277–280, 1988.

Smith, Everett L., and Catherine Gilligan. "Physical Activity Effects on Bone Metabolism." *Calcified Tissue International.* 49:S50–S54, 1991.

Smith, Everett L., Catherine Gilligan, Marianne McAdam, Cynthia P. Ensign, and Patricia E. Smith. "Deterring Bone Loss by Exercise Intervention in Premenopausal and Postmenopausal Women." *Calcified Tissue International.* 44:312–321, 1989.

Spilner, Maggie. *Prevention's Complete Book of Walking.* Emmaus, PA: Rodale, Inc., 2000.

Todd, Mabel E. *The Thinking Body.* Hightstown, NJ: Princeton Book Company, 1968.

Westcott, Wayne L. "Muscular Strength and Endurance." In *Personal Trainer Manual: The Resource for Fitness Instructors.* Mitchell Study (ed.), Boston, MA: Reebok University Press. 235–274, 1996.

Westcott, Wayne. *Building Strength and Stamina.* Champaign, IL: Human Kinetics, 1996.

Westcott, Wayne. *Strength Fitness,* 3rd Edition. Dubuque, IA: William C. Brown Publishers, 1991.

Westcott, W.S. *Strength Fitness: Physiological Principles and Training Techniques,* 4th Edition. Dubuque, IA: William C. Brown Publishers, 1995.

Yanker, Gary, and Kathy Burton. *Walking Medicine.* New York: McGraw-Hill, 1993.

Index

A

abdominal exercises, and Fitness Walking Plus, 25–27; and form, 68; and Strength Training, 50–54; and Target Toning, 67–71

abdominal muscle groups, 25–27, 67–68

accessibility of Fitness Walking, 4

aerobic activity, 24, 97

aging, 7, 97–98

alternatives to Fitness Walking, 88–90

American College of Sports Medicine, *xiii*, 18, 21

arm exercises, and Fitness Walking Plus, 32–34; and Strength Training, 56–57; and Target Toning, 80–82

arm movements (in Fitness Walking), 13

B

back exercises, 58

back-of-thigh and buns toner, 48–49

bands, resistance, 6, 33–34, 38

baseline walking fitness level, 17

bent-over arm raise, 58

biceps curls, 56

blisters, 11

body shape, 4; changing, 5–6, 24

bone density, 6–7

boredom, 96–97

breakfast, importance of, 96

breathing, 14, 37

buttocks exercises, and Fitness Walking Plus, 27–29; and Strength Training, 48–49; and Target Toning, 78–79

C

calendar, 94

calf stretch, 20

calorie burning, 5, 95

cellulite, 25

clothing, 11–12

cold weather walking, 11–12

cool down, 14

CoolMax, 11

D

diagonal abdominals, 52–53

diagonal/side abdominal toners, 71

diet, 25, 95–96

doctor's approval for walking, 10

dress, 11–12

Dri-FIT, 11

duration of exercise, 17, 18

E

equipment, 2, 6, 10; resistance bands, 33–34; for Strength Training, 38; treadmill, 17

Index

exercise repetitions, 37–38

exercise sets, 37–38

exercises, abdominal, 50–55, 67–71, 101; back, 58; buttocks, 27–29; 48–49; 78–79; heel raise—toe raise, 40–41; overview, 100–110; thigh, 29–32; 42–49, 72–77; upper arms, 32–34; 56–57, 80–82

F

fat, 24–25, 36

feet, care of , 10–11; and proper walking technique, 13

15-Minute Strength Training Program, 39, 59–61

Fitness Walking, 2, 3, 9–22, 111; and aging, 97–98; baseline level, 17; as cardiovascular exercise, 15–16, 113–114; creating a walking program, 17–19; and equipment, 10–12; finding your baseline walking fitness level, 17; frequency, 86; goals, 22, 86; and hydration, 21–22; posture, 12–13; and safety, 22; and stretching, 19–21; and the target zone, 14–16; technique, 12–13

Fitness Walking Plus, 2, 3, 5–6, 23–34, 95, 111; abdominal muscles, 25–27, 101; buttocks toning, 27–29; frequency, 86; goals, 86; thighs, 29–32; upper arms, 32–34

flexibility, 19–21. *See also* stretching

fluid intake, 21–22, 95

food journal, 96

food shopping, 96

form, 5, 19; in abdominal exercises, 68; in buttocks tightener, 78; in Fitness Walking, 5, 12–13, 100; in Strength Training, 36; in Target Toning, 67

frequency of exercise, Fitness Walking, 18, 86; Strength Training, 38, 87; Target Toning, 67, 68, 87

front-thigh toner, 72–74

G

Gamex, 12

goal setting, 17–18, 22

Gore-Tex, 12

H

hamstring stretch, 21

heart rate, 5, 14, 15–16, 113–114

heart-rate monitor, 16

heel raise—toe raise, 40–41

hill walking, 19, 31–32, 95

hip stretch, 20

hot weather walking, 11

housework, 88–90

hydration, 21–22, 95

I

impact of walking, 4

indoor exercise, housework, 88–90; treadmill, 17

inner-thigh toner, 46–47, 76–77

intensity of walking, 5, 14–16, 95

Index

substitutions for Fitness Walking, 88–90

sunscreen, 11

supplies, 2, 6, 10; resistance bands, 33–34; for strength training, 38; treadmill, 17

Surgeon General's Report on Physical Activity and Health (1996), *xiii*

T

taking your pulse, 15–16, 113–114

talk test, 14

Target Toning, 2, 3, 6, 7, 63–84, 111–112; abdomen, 67–71; and aging, 97–98; buttocks, 78–79; exercises, 66, 106–110; frequency, 87; goals, 87; guidelines, 66, 68, 78, 80; inventory, 65; needs, 64; posture, 67; scheduling, 67; stretching, 80, 83; thighs, 72–77; upper arms, 80–82

target zone, heart rate, 5, 14–16, 113–114; perceived exertion, 14–15; talk test, 14

ten-second target zone, 16, 114

thigh exercises, and Fitness Walking Plus, 29–32; and Strength Training, 42–49; and Target Toning, 72–77

thigh stretch, 20

Thinsulate, 12

Thintech, 12

30-Minute Strength Training Program, 39, 40–58

treadmills, 17

triceps extension, 57

U

upper-abdominal toners, 50–51, 69

upper-arm toners, 81–82

V

vegetables, 96

Versatech, 12

W

walking duration, 17

walking shoes, 10–11

warm up, 14, 36

water intake, 21–22, 95

weather, 11–12

weekly exercise plans, 85–98, 112

weight loss, 4, 5, 6, 24–25, 95

weights, 6, 22, 38

wind, walking in, 12

worksheets, 115–119

Y

yardwork, 88–90